The Most Unhealthy Relationship Of All

Other Books by Mark Hertzberg

Memories of Tomorrow: The Adventures of Comicman

And Forthcoming in 2,003

Improvisation and Standup Comedy techniques for everyday life.

The Most Unhealthy Relationship Of All

✦

A Guide To Better Doctor–Patient Communication

by

Dr. Mark A Hertzberg

Steve Bedney, Editor

iUniverse, Inc.
New York Lincoln Shanghai

The Most Unhealthy Relationship Of All
A Guide To Better Doctor–Patient Communication

iUniverse, Inc.

For information address:
iUniverse, Inc.
2021 Pine Lake Road, Suite 100
Lincoln, NE 68512
www.iuniverse.com

ISBN: 0-595-27200-2

Printed in the United States of America

Two Reasons

Anyone who knows me sees this book as the predictable result of my gift for gab. Of course I talk more to patients than any other doctor would, so why wouldn't I write about communication in the doctor's office? They do not guess at the other half of the puzzle: I easily pick up on what so many doctors and patients do wrong because, naturally, I do them right!

That last point was not meant as a joke. Long before I had any degrees I was able to get doctors to speak clearly and to explain completely. Granted, I was lucky enough to start with some fantastic doctors. It is possible that this led me to expect smooth communications, and that can only have helped. I do not believe the fact that I could grasp concepts very quickly had that much to do with it, although I would like to believe that my charming and fascinating personality helped. The truth is, I did everything right because I was trained.

Luck is the residue of design. I started out with fantastic doctors because my parents picked fantastic doctors. My parents also had a certain standing in the community. That might have made it easier for them to make themselves known to these doctors, but, ultimately, the doctors would get to know them and that determined their relationships with these doctors. In fact, it was their lack of ever trying to act like they had a special position that was their greatest communication tool. You get more respect by showing some than by demanding some.

My mother is the queen of preparation. If she says she'll have something done by a certain time, you can set your watch to it. If I had an appointment to see the doctor, she'd figure on getting there on time to fill out forms and take care of any unforseen technicalities. She'd leave plenty of time in case we were delayed in traffic, or had a flat tire. If the doctor gave her instructions she made certain that she understood them and had the important things written down. If she was uncertain of something she would ask if it was okay if my father phoned later. She'd even ask if there was a best time for such a call when it wouldn't interfere with the doctor's hectic schedule. Because the doctors knew my parents would be respectful of their time, they generally said that anytime would be fine.

With medical treatment, and in fact with any consumer issue, my mother has a simple rule that she uses to incredible benefit: It never hurts to ask. The specifics of this plan are fiendishly simple. Always be polite, be persistent if you must, but only if you must, and act grateful even if you feel entitled.

The first time I was allowed to ride my bike to a dental appointment my mother called down to tell me it was time to get ready. I already had my coat on. Without any lectures or courses I had been trained to take responsibility for my own health care, and that has always "naturally" been appreciated by my doctors.

My father eventually added "hospital chaplain" to his resume'. Long before this, he had become well known in local (New York City and Long Island) medical circles. He would talk to doctors on behalf of some patients, and he'd talk to patients to assist some doctors. What really stood out is when doctors called upon him to talk to other doctors. I recall one case when a doctor felt a patient absolutely had to be admitted to another hospital because of the excellence of a certain department. As the doctor put it to my father, nobody can get in there, so I came to you. My father has never had any actual political or industrial power, but he seems to be able to speak to everybody. He also has a sixth sense for navigating through bureaucracies. It may have taken many phone calls and an in-person stop-by or two, but he got a foot in the door for this patient.

To me, such communication seemed normal. Later I learned how extraordinary it was. It would never occur to me to throw up my hands in frustration when communication seems impossible, because I know it is possible. I know the problems are not just because doctors won't talk to patients, but, rather, because both doctors and patients have many problems adding up to the big problem. And I knew, as in the case of this doctor who called my father on behalf of his patient, that just because a doctor may not be the great communicator does not mean the doctor isn't going all out for the patient.

This book is actually the result of observing doctors and patients trying all sorts of things while I knew the keys to opening the lines of communication were so simple. The two reasons it exists are my first two teachers, so this book is dedicated to them.

To Mom and Dad

Like everything else, good doctor–patient
communication begins at home.

Contents

Special Thanks

For my first book I went out a got a "hired gun" to edit my manuscript—not an easy task considering the experimental style of that project. We became friends which is good—I couldn't put a price on help he gave me with this book.

To
Steve Bedney

Explanation of Special Terms

He or She?

Surprise. You will not need a medical dictionary to read this book. There is no good reason that things can't be explained in regular words. There is, however, one big word problem. Despite my attempts to change things, English still insists on separate pronouns for males and females and has no generic option. Even if I flipped a coin each time to choose between 'he' or 'she,' people would still read into each choice. No matter how a reader tried to avoid it, the pronoun used carries a nuance.

Until I can officially update the English language, or my editor accepts 'they' and 'them' as singular, here is my personal solution. Whenever a chance for a generic pronoun arises, you will see h/s or h/h. These stand for he or she, his or her, and him or her. You can read them as male, female, both, either or something in between.

Prologue
I was a Nuclear Optometrist

In 1982 I was just a student with no inkling of the incredible savvy I would one day pretend to have. On arriving to start a two week assignment at a VA center on Long Island my friend and I passed a sign, "NUCLEAR MEDICINE." Wow. Talk about impressive. Fortunately I remained cool enough to immediately point out that this was a typo, the U and the N were switched. I then made a proper sign, "Unclear Medicine."

The great thing about that sign was that you could put it anywhere. No matter what specialty you speak of, people find this title to be appropriate. It's the one-size-fits-all of titles. I invented and declared myself the world's foremost expert in the field of "Nuclear," excuse me, "Unclear Optometry." After twenty years of finding this title to be perfect I have taken a new challenge: Make some little bit of health care, somewhere, somehow, not fit into this heretofore infinite category. And to do that I might have to stop using words like "heretofore."

Let me make one thing perfectly clear. A lot of medical stuff is complicated. Very complicated. Far beyond the comprehension of most people. Most doctors are people. Most of them are confused too. I am told that some people stop talking when they aren't sure what to say.[1] You are reading this book because you think you want to get your doctor over this. If you succeeded you'd hear uncertainty in your doctor's voice on occasion. This might lead to your running to the streets screaming something like, "The end is near."[2] You're probably best off treating your medical care like walking off a cliff in a cartoon: Don't

---

1. It's an option that has never occurred to me, but I am told about it.
2. If you're still in that hospital gown this will take on a completely new meaning.

look down and you won't fall. You've just finished all you need from this book; the rest is just filler to make it thick enough. If you insist on being stubborn about trying to communicate, read on at your own peril.

Dr. Doolittle spent all that time learning the languages of the animals only to use it to throw medical jargon at them. Some doctors plain can't communicate. To make matters worse, some patients can't either. As a patient you might be fed up with trying to communicate with doctors. Believe it or not, many doctors are at the ends of their ropes trying to deal with patients.

Some doctors talk funny for reasons, but I guess that's fair since some patients come in playing their own games. Lots of patients have communication strategies to get the doctor to speak differently, while that very doctor may be devising methods of getting that patient to provide the right information. Then both sides counter defensively so that any strategies planned to open the lines of communication back-fire. Got it? I didn't think so. Okay, sit down, get a snack, let's talk.

I did not do any scientific research into the communication habits of millions of health care professionals to put this book together. If you disagree with anything just take it as food for thought. I'm in my comedy/novel writing office now, not in a clinic; If you don't like what I write, don't laugh. Calling a malpractice attorney will do you no good since being the first comedian sued for such would be a great help to my career. With that disclaimer out of the way, I will say that I do believe I know what I am talking about.

I never spend a day in the exam room without at least one patient saying that h/s wished other doctors would work with h/h as I do. I have rarely gone through a day without at least one patient saying my exam was the best h/s's ever had by any type of doctor, ever. Many patients ask me to help with conditions completely out of my field because h/s can't get that doctor to explain something or to understand something. The truth is I could be giving a totally incompetent exam and few patients would know. The only patients who can be sure I did a great job are those who had lifetime problems that nobody could solve until they came to my exam room. All the others are just reacting to the fact that I talk a lot.

As the most talkative doctor—okay, the most talkative *anything*—on the planet I have always been keenly aware of what patients do in my exam room and how this relates to our communication. Since I am always asked why other doctors don't talk like I do, I have always looked at everything from that perspective: How would a normal person[3] react to what patients do? Few people, doctors or otherwise, would keep talking when faced with things I deal with regularly. Everything that follows is based on two decades of these observations, mixed with some observations of other doctors, nurses, PAs, and administrators I have worked with, as well as a few I have spoken to as friends. I even made a few observations you might label as "undercover work": I played the role of patient! Unless I am specifically asked I never tell a doctor examining me what I do, so do not think for a moment that I am treated differently.

Since long before I started playing doctor I have been a comedian. Obviously, comedic ability should be required for every job involving interaction with people (or with anything else), but it should be more than a supplement when doctoring. At the core, good doctoring and good comedy rely on the same skills! Here's an inside secret: It doesn't take brilliance to acquire all the knowledge required to pass tests of medical skill. In fact, being a bit dull helps when it comes to memorizing reams of boring facts, names, and statistics. Real associative intellect—the kind used to create a snappy reply in an instant—is more important for dealing with medical diagnoses in the real world. There's no time to list 11,000 obscure possibilities a straight-A-student-drone has memorized. It's critical to pull out the few that count instantly. When a patient presents a twist on anything covered by any book, the special doctor is the one able to associate the possibilities creatively.

---

3.   In this case "normal" can be defined as having the ability I lack to stop talking.

This ability to make creative associations is what you call "clever" in a comedian.

Comedic ability also helps with the communication itself. Personally, I work in a manner that few doctors would find comfortable. I am not advising anyone to work exactly as I do: I am a professional, do not try this in your office. On the other hand I keep the power of humor in mind when I am cast in the role of patient, and that always helps. On both sides it has helped me figure out what is happening when things go wrong. Just like we are told by relationship counselors that when *he says "X" he means "X" but she hears "Y" and vice versa,* doctors and patients often use the same basic words and come up with very different understandings.

If you would be so gracious as to indulge me for a moment, I would like to tell you something about my view of humor. Don't worry, this will be short; otherwise, there would be no use in buying other books from me on this topic.

We always talk about a *sense of humor,* but nobody questions what this means. Finding something to be funny is not a sense. You sense something by seeing, hearing, touching, smelling, or tasting. You may judge it to be funny, but you don't really *sense* the funny in it. You may rearrange details to produce humor from a topic, but if we weren't trained to call this ability a sense we never would make the mistake of doing so. Someone who laughs at everything does not have a great sense of humor anymore than someone who sees mirages and hears voices has great vision and hearing. Someone who tells lots of jokes doesn't necessarily have a great sense of humor, but h/s probably does have more need for attention than ability to earn it. Making jokes[4] is not a sense; neither is laughing at everything.

---

4.   Timing itself can arguably be labeled a sense. It definitely is when you adjust the timing in a one-on-one situation to make that one person laugh. When dealing with large groups or written humor it may imply a sense of some timing that works generally, for most people.

My personal take is that maybe somebody who knew something very profound coined the phrase "sense of humor" and everyone else is just playing the game of telephone with this phrase. The sense part is the ability to sense what will make another person laugh! It is a very deep interpersonal skill. It is easy to guess that a gun or a rabid wolf might scare you, that a winning lottery ticket might bring some joy to you, or even that the winning ticket might make you depressed if you are that type of negative person. It is hard to figure out what will make anyone laugh. Your oldest friend will sometimes surprise you when h/s does or doesn't laugh, yet people try to make strangers laugh. Put me at a dinner table with someone and I will get them laughing no matter how rarely they laugh and how much they despise my attempts to be funny. I sense things about each action and reaction and find my way. I believe I am uncovering the core of their psyches, but there is no need to get so grandiose about things here.

Thank you for your kind indulgence. We now understand that we posses an ability to sense something of the inner workings of people. The goal of using this ability does not have to be laughter—we have use for much easier levels. Honing these abilities is a topic for another time. Fortunately, in the upcoming chapter we have lots of inside stuff concerning what's going on in your doctor's head, prepackaged for your convenience…

1

Why Dr. Johnny Can't Speak

People ask why doctors talk "that way" all the time. What way? Granted, some doctors talk funny, but "that way" can be many different things. Some people are asking about haughty doctors; some about cold ones. There are also technical ones, jargon-dependent ones, rushed ones, secretive ones, and otherwise fantastic ones who can't get the point across.

Sooner or later a doctor must use technical words, but sometimes avoiding them causes problems. There can be a nuance to a doctor's voice that seems condescending when taken to mean, "I'm using simple words even you can understand." From some doctors, however, this tone is actually the medical equivalent of, *look ma, no hands!* They are saying, "hey, look, no technical jargon, so don't go saying I tried to confuse you."

There are many different styles of "that way," and many different reasons for them. Doctors have to deal with many patients. Whatever way your doctor speaks to you is affected by all of these other patients. Generally, patients do many things incorrectly when it comes to health and medical care. For instance, brushing my teeth a hundred times the week before a dental check up does not make up for years of neglect. Trying to hide things in this manner can be a problem when providing facts needed for a diagnosis. People try to steer the facts toward what they guess is a safe answer: *This heartburn was a little more than average, they told me when I regained consciousness, so I agreed to have you check my heartburn just to be safe.*

When a patient's own tension causes problems, h/s may defensively create stories about the doctor's attitude. Every reader of this book has a collection of anecdotes told by friends and acquaintances. As with stories of any type, the truth is probably somewhat different. The better sounding the story, the further from the truth it may have moved.

Exaggerated stories cause fears of bad working relationships that become self-fulfilling prophecies. Once we understand this we can make sure we don't take an adversarial view of the medical practitioner. The vast majority are working harder to keep patients healthy than most patients are doing for themselves. Team up with them. If they have problems communicating, work with them on that too.

◆   ◆   ◆

Like "regular people," many doctors like hearing their own voice. It's maybe the top thing to hear other than the sound of one's own name, which gets a star added if there's a title included. There are people who need such reinforcement so much, they become doctors just for the title. Some people's favorite thing to hear is their own special "pomp and circumstance" voice, dolled out in small allowances. This explains why some people become doctors or judges or politicians. Or cult leaders. Or, worse, radio talk show hosts. Or public speakers like myself.

To save time some doctors replace long monologues with short "soliloquies," complete with ego-fulfilling-Shakespearian tones—even a metered delivery! Let them have their fun. Don't confuse getting the information you want with getting them to speak the way you want.

Let's say you have a humble doctor. When talking about last night's ballgame h/s can communicate like anyone else. This makes you go ballistic inside when it's time to discuss your condition and h/s starts speaking in tongues. You may wonder, "What is h/s hiding?" Actually, h/s has several possibilities to choose from.

You want the truth? You can't handle the truth!

To understand Dr. Johnny[1] let's go back and see how h/s got to be the way h/s is. There is no magic moment when Student Johnny or Intern Johnny becomes Dr. Johnny. Student Johnny begins to realize that although h/s is accumulating facts, h/s is still just Johnny; H/s is not methodically changing into a magical entity.

That's just about as likely to happen as anybody one day realizing h/s is a total, "accredited" parent. One day you are technically a parent because you have kids, but no fairy-god-parent came with a wand and truly turned you into one. You just improvise your way, hoping your cover is never broken, hoping your kids survive the fact that you are just an older kid pretending to act like Grandma and Grandpa did.

Similarly, a med student just feels h/h way along until graduation. There's a ceremony where a Wizard-of-Oz wannabe hands out papers. "Back in Kansas there are people with no more healing powers than you have. But they have something you don't—A diploma! And a license." After years of handling thousands of cases h/s may feel like h/s's truly a doctor; however, h/h style had set in during the early stages.

I prefer a doctor who feels like a bit of an impostor. The other option is one who feels no awe at the responsibility of having people's lives in h/h hands, working with only our still-limited medical knowledge, which is far beyond what any one human can grasp anyway!

You don't want a doctor who felt no terror when h/s first realized how impossibly large the totality of medical knowledge is. Any student who figured, "it's the same for all doctors, patients have to live with this reality," is dangerous. Patients die with this reality. Give me the doctor who does everything possible to get around the reality of h/h limitations. I don't mind a doctor at peace with h/h limitations. I don't mind a doctor who is proud of h/h superiority to other doctors. I will

---

1.   You are of course aware that this can also be pronounced Dr. Joanie in Ye elde English.

have nothing to do with a doctor who is dismissive of the fact of limitations.

You might guess that anyone who feels no awe or proper responsibility in being a doctor is in it for the money. Being in it for the money is not a problem by itself. Many people pick medicine for the money but wrestle with the decision: *To earn the right to earn the money requires a supreme effort.* There are years of suffering to learn instead of already having a salary and hanging out with the buds. Think about those years of fun and freedom when you had a job and spending money, but no spouse or kids yet. The vast majority of doctors sacrificed those years entirely.

There are some doctors spending their careers in Peace Corp—like settings, but there is no reliable source of saints to stock the med schools. Most people wouldn't go through what doctors go through even for the money. For those who do, money is part of it. Accept that and move on.

So, doctors are regular people who never magically transformed. How do you think it seems to them when the first thing anyone ever says about them is that they are doctors? At a party you wouldn't introduce someone as Grocer Jim or Sanitation Woman Jill or Accountant Stan, but you would introduce your friend as Dr. Alex. Jim works as a grocer, it isn't what he is—unless he insists on that. He may think of himself as theater afficionado Jim, or Family Jim. You think of Alex as doctor. It's not his job, it's not even his career, it's what he is! Only a small percentage of doctors think that way—maybe not that much different than grocers. If everyone thought of Alex as Alex, a guy with some medical training, it wouldn't be so hard to deal with the fact that deep down Alex knows he was never magically transformed into a doctor.

People are upset that doctors don't act more human, but people won't forgive doctors the moment they dare act human. Is it any wonder that some doctors talk "that way" to be protective of what they don't know?

Another reason some doctors talk "that way" is to save time. Use a few big words that represent entire topics and voila', the whole explanation has officially been given. For extra protection hit the patient with a tone of *don't look like a dummy by saying you don't understand this.* This works even better with patients who want to feel they've done their share, but have no desire to make a real effort to understand a good explanation.

Ease of (alleged) comprehension is why people like numbers.[2] Tell a patient that the condition h/s came in with is vision of "twenty fifty" so h/s's getting glasses and you make h/h, h/h insurance company, employer, motor vehicle bureau, and everyone else including yourself happy. The fact that such a diagnosis/explanation is actually meaningless drivel is beside the point.

You know what happens when you use a couple of big words? People keep quiet. When I explain with simple words the complainers see an opening. They'll always include an accusation that I used big words, but they can never point any out. The only word anyone has even tried to name is "unit" (of power for the glasses prescription).

If I say "diopter" then they really don't understand. Nobody has ever asked me to explain what a diopter is. Maybe they just get the message that it isn't intended for them to understand. When I keep it simple I get attacked 5 or 6 % of the time: "What the hell is a unit, stop confusing things with big words." I point out that "unit" is not a technical word, I avoided the actual term "diopter" so they wouldn't need to study optics to understand it. All that counts is there is some kind of unit of this and we are discussing a certain amount of them.

---

2.   I recently read an essay about the general fear and avoidance of numbers. It's undeniable. However, there can be a rebound effect. People overrate numbers because of fear. This fear makes numbers seem substantial enough to replace an entire explanation. Due to this fear few people ask to have the numbers explained. This lets their lack of real meaning stay secret.

The upshot is, the easiest way to eliminate these annoyances involves confusing everybody with big words. By keeping people quiet time is saved.

Anytime a doctor talks it may become a conversation. H/s may not be able to end it so h/s must make it clear that it is a one way lecture. Given the chance, nearly every patient will try to talk for several exam slots but few would agree to pay to cover several exams. So, doctors talk haughtily and you get the message to listen.

By the way, when it comes to really good explanations, even teachers in medical schools have trouble getting the truly complex things across very well. These things are very complicated, and even doctors don't have enough "brain RAM[3]" to handle the details. Maybe back in med school in some shining moment of supreme clarity while cramming they really grasped the entire concept at hand, but they probably couldn't keep hold of it long enough to help the next guy in the study group through. They certainly don't know every concept well enough to teach it years later. They feel good about themselves for mastering enough to use the great storehouse of knowledge. No one person will ever be the great storehouse of knowledge.

Dr. Hyde and Mr. Jekyl
(Yes, the names are reversed)

A doctor needs a special nature to survive—a marvelous balance of sensitivity and detachment. Detachment is a special kind of insensitivity. See how problems might arise? Having seen doctors develop I have realized that many actually create characters to be the doctors. I'd wager few realize it, but they really are a different person, one who can deal with stuff that would floor h/h normal self. You got it—Dr. Hyde.

---

3.   Computers make this concept easier to grasp. Even with tons (gigabytes) of knowledge only a drop can be consciously handled (Ks of RAM) at once. And you need to consult the web for the real storehouse of knowledge.

Most doctor and nurse candidates are less squeamish than the average person. I was not. Many things I see on the job don't even arouse the attention of my *squeamish sensors,* but I never became equivalently numb to such things outside of the office. The character I am on the job has no access to the squeamish function. He uses no will power because the concept of being conscious of the disgusting nature of things just doesn't exist for him.[4] If I step out of the office and see something a tenth as disgusting, an aversion reflex kicks in loud and clear.

It isn't really being distant; it's more like being so close you don't see anything but individual pieces of information. It's like a digital forest where you can only be aware of the information defining one tree at a time. The disgusting stuff requires putting it all together and seeing the forest. I don't see an injured person with a horrifying swollen eye with blood and pus and—you get the picture. Well, I don't. I see little pipes up close leaking a nice shade of scarlet liquid onto a canvas white background with…*Just the facts ma'am.* If a similar case walks into a restaurant and sits across from me, *ooo icch, feeling, nauseated, appetite gone,…*

Any lack of conversation by a doctor is confused with coldness; however, if h/s doesn't maintain a certain distance as if on some level you are an object, then h/s'd have a psychological meltdown at a very young age. I believe humor is very helpful here, but that's not for now. Some actual coldness also helps detail work be more objective. Many patients are actually reassured by a certain aloof coldness from their physician. Warmth makes a doctor seem more like a friend, but maybe less like someone with the power to make you recover.

Some patients want their doctor to act like god; an omnipotent attitude can be very reassuring. Any understanding on their own part demystifies the process, depriving them of the faith in the magic nature of their doctor that they require to help recover.

---

4.   He does notice the awful odors of some patients

Coldness or distance also prevents a patient from getting too clingy. Clingy patients who feel they have a nice, warm, cuddly doctor feel comfortable asking questions to which they really don't want the answer.

We are boldly going where no doctor or patient has gone before, so let's get a perspective on the route we are exploring.

Super Secret Hint

Here's the book's big surprise ending a bit early. To understand each other realize that there is no intrinsic difference. This is how you'd behave if circumstances were switched. Think of how best to deal with yourself in such circumstances and everything else will fall into place.

Doctors do not come from some mystical doctor tribe; they start out the same as everyone else. Like regular people, most doctors would rather talk than have an awkward silence. So why would they evolve a pattern of causing such silences? Actually, many who try to, can't. Some doctors who you think are silent actually banter more than you realize.

We are always aware of our dentist's banter because of our trouble responding. Of course the dentist has time to banter while h/s works on you. If you drill teeth all the time it becomes mindless physical work except for occasional moments of checking things. During these moments your dentist drops out of the conversation, then rejoins the conversation already in progress. Surgeons probably do likewise, but with any luck you're unconscious at the time. Most of the time that you spend with a medical doctor you are being checked. H/s is absorbing information rather than performing a "mindless" procedure. H/s has to spend a higher percentage of this time concentrating.

In the case of doctors who are the "strong silent types," or with all doctors who have periods of such silence, the best way to open the channels of communication is to get inside h/h head. To lure someone out of a self-imposed awkward silence consider what would make you yourself learn to prefer it in the first place.

First you'd come up with our explanation of needing to concentrate. As a doctor you would have much more on your mind than, let's say, a mechanic, who is not interrupted by the car to explain what h/s's doing. For a homework experiment try to stay with a mechanic for the entire time that h/s works on your car to discuss what's happening. Demand explanations and challenge what h/s's doing. Good luck. You'll be visiting a doctor in short time.

Stepping into the doctor's shoes you may wonder if less talkative people pick these shoes more often. Maybe. It is my observation that the system used to filter med school candidates favors some of the worst ones by its ill-conceived design. It favors somewhat robotic (dull?) people; not brilliant original thinkers, social butterflies, nor great communicators.

One has to memorize tons of boring facts to display "intelligence" to the system. An intelligent person with social skills wouldn't have enough time to sit alone memorizing, and would get too bored anyway. A certain lack of intelligence is an advantage to memorize thoughtlessly and spit things back verbatim like a tape recorder. True understanding requires thinking about things. Such thought always shows up as an imperfect playback of the listed facts. Many of the listed facts are outdated or are plain mistakes. With a little thought it's apparent these don't fit in with other things you've learned. If you have the intellect to figure that out and this affects your answers for the better, it will affect your grades for the worse!

Another reason you might keep quiet in a doctor's shoes is that the conversation is monotonous. The excitement level of a medical exam is very different from the other side of the stethoscope. When it comes to discussing things that may seem earthshaking to you, to the doctor it's the thirtieth time h/s's had to deal with the same completely routine thing this week. And it's only Tuesday. Routine cases are dull to explain, and saying, "trust me, this is a routine thing," doesn't cut it.

Once you've worn the doctor's shoes through years of schooling and practice you may no longer be able to relate to the basic levels needed to explain things. A doctor may not grasp what it is a patient doesn't understand (there's a pun in there somewhere). Let's try to make this a bit more academic...

In college, classes may have thousands of students under some impressive professor. H/s answers questions by missing their point entirely or by assuming a knowledge base that these students couldn't attain for years. Without that knowledge students can't "decode" the professor's reply. Ask the same question to the grad student assisting the professor and you get a great answer. The grad student remembers how much h/s did not know a few years ago. H/s takes the question at face value and answers to fill the gaps in your knowledge.

So, if you come in with routine conditions, the doctor is bored and can't relate to your level anyway; but, if you come in with something complex, it requires h/h full attention and is too hard to explain anyway. Beside, h/s may be nervous about saying too much.

Explaining is an art. It requires a deeper understanding than is required simply to use the knowledge. When I tutored (pre) med students in basic physics I discovered something: They preferred to ignore understanding in lieu of thoughtless memorization. This works fine when memorizing the bones of animals in comparative anatomy. As discussed earlier this is easier for dullards than for geniuses.[5] Einstein refused to waste time and brain space memorizing such things. He even refused to memorize constants in physics. To quote him to the

---

5.   The screening processes of all fields favor memorizers over deep thinkers. They talk about wanting brilliant thinkers who will advance the knowledge of the field, but those in charge are concerned that nobody challenges the status quo that has them in power. Admission to any kind of school screens out rebels in favor of those who toe the party line. Geniuses must pretend to agree to qualify as intelligent enough. Many can't or won't. Einstein was not accepted anywhere until after he became a "superstar" on his own.

best of my recall, "why would I waste time memorizing something I can easily look up?"[6] [7]

There are certain courses of extra interest to an individual med student that h/s does understand in great depth. There are also some graduates who have no great understanding of anything. Some of these make fine, mechanical, doctors. Even the most outstanding med student of all time who had a deep comprehension of everything in school will lose most of it. Ten years later "superstudent" would be lucky to retain detailed comprehension of 10%. H/s may have a workable knowledge of two or three times that depending on the scope of h/h practice. The bigger a specialist h/s is, the less broad h/h scope. The specialist has great depth of knowledge (we hope) on a fraction of a percent.

A lot of what is taught in school never comes up for any given doctor. Some of it is useful only to medical research scientists. A lot of it never comes up for anyone. Sometimes, it's there because the people who teach it lobbied to get it required by the state. Even if we could cut med school down to just real usable medical knowledge, the last time a human being could have had a good grasp of all "Western" medical knowledge was over a century ago.

I have seen statistics that claim total medical knowledge doubles every two to three years. This stat existed even before the widespread use of computers and other high-tech assists to advancing research. You never know what a stat really means when you only hear the stat itself, so let's assume this total knowledge includes drivel. Let's make

---

6.   Okay, it was probably more like "vy voote I vaste…"

7.   Remember this desire for lists of facts over depth of understanding. It will help us understand another level of the "dehumanizing" way doctors sometimes view patients. The more complicated things become the more the clarity of a list and maybe some numerical values is desired. To keep your condition clear in h/h mind it, and by extension you, may become more and more a list of facts. Catch 22: The worse your medical condition, the more you want the human touch, but the worse the condition, the less the doctor may be able to give. Too bad we can't just give h/h brain more RAM at the time.

allowance for things like lists of identical pharmaceutical products by competing firms, slightly different variants, and even packaging details. Maybe the real knowledge was possible to master 80 years ago and it doesn't double quite so quickly, so let's be conservative and say it doubles every 8 years. It has doubled 10 times in 80 years. That's 1024 times the knowledge one human might master. Good thing we kept conservative.

Your doctor has to be a wizard just to know where to look things up and with whom to consult. But h/s can't drop the facade, or you'd be terrified and run out screaming. So the facade must stay: *Ignore that feeble minded human behind the curtain, I am the great and powerful "Physician of OZ."* Silence is often the easiest way to keep up the act. And the perceived rudeness of haughty origin actually helps sell the act.

Some doctors can be very good despite very little deep comprehension. They can't explain in depth because that's past the point where they truly understand, and far past the point where they can really explain. This can actually be the foundation of their good performance because they know what to do and are clear headed. They don't bog down on theory and wonder if they should fine tune every little procedural detail. They can follow directions to a cure like you can turn on all the components of a very sophisticated home entertainment system.[8] You don't have to understand how a single component works.

Compare this with pilots. They have to demonstrate some familiarity with what keeps the plane up, but the science doesn't really come up often while flying. They know the moves. They don't bog down thinking how each thing scientifically works in order to choose which move to make. If the movies are correct, then test pilots are different. They think in terms of what has to be changed with an experimental craft as they fly it. They think like scientists and engineers so they can discuss things with the engineers. There are doctors on the forefront who are like this; a combination of real-time practitioner with the

---

8.   Don't worry if you need your kids to help you: The doctor may have kids to help
      with the more modern equipment.

mind of a researcher. Yes they exist, but how often is *Chuck Yeager* piloting your flight to Miami?

We see that expertise is a matter of degree. The true experts design things. A genius devises theories behind such designs. Those who operate or fix things need less expertise, if any. For some hiding this gets nasty: They make you resent that you are not an expert by implying you could not understand it.

I figure that styles set in early. Back then the young clinician was more concerned about wether h/s'd survive giving a medical examination while being observed and having to answer a supervisor's quizzes. H/s would never want to encourage a patient to ask tougher questions. H/s had to display a good bedside manner, but at the same time steer the conversation to safe, easy questions. Possibly without realizing it, young interns learn to seem pleasant while preventing a real exchange of information.

Lots[9] of doctors are unaware of their actual style of conversation and why it is that way, but likely it developed back when they had supervisors over their shoulders. It was further molded when they were first on their own and probably very nervous.

◆   ◆   ◆

When going for a dramatic effect, big words build on what silence starts. It's also easier to remember big words than the complete big concept behind each. A doctor just has to remember that a standard treatment goes with this big word, which h/s can look up. You can't look up a concept.

---

9.   This is simply my observation. My editor is of the opinion that I should not have the words "I think" at the start of this sentence because people are supposed to understand that many things stated are simply my opinion. He does not, however, mind this footnote because it mentions him.

◆   ◆   ◆

Here's another reason a doctor might keep quiet. Malingerers[10] look for clues to guide them as they fake things. Talk from the doctor is used as a source of clues to help them adjust. Malingerers quickly train doctors to say "no" more than necessary.

Speaking of saying "no" more, yes, there are secrets being kept. Do you know how a cold is diagnosed? You come with symptoms like a cold so you are treated for a cold. The treatment is the test. The other choice is to spend huge sums of money on testing that would give a definitive answer too late to be useful anyway. If yours doesn't run the normal course you are treated as the next most likely thing at the time. If the usual suspects are all accounted for, then you go for expensive, sophisticated testing. The millions of people who have a cold don't want to be told, "Looks like a cold, but it's not possible to be sure."

◆   ◆   ◆

If a doctor does converse h/s likes the patient to get to the point briefly. Once started many patients will keep adding nonsequiturs and search for more questions.[11] They feel the doctor must listen, so any story has a captive audience. A doctor who has permitted talk will also hear about other doctors who won't listen. Because h/s is presently struggling to get back to work h/s does not take this as a compliment, but as advice to become like those doctors.

At some level patients who realize they've found that great talking doctor react in the worst way: Instead of finding out how to get other doctors to talk, the easier solution is to make this doctor cover for them

---

10.   The less technical word is "fakers." Also liars, cheats, con artists.

11.   In two decades I have never heard a last question. Last statements are also rare, except for, *I have to run and feed the meter.* If I am unable to conclude instantly I am doomed, for if I allow h/h back into the office h/s feels h/s's paid for the next hour.

all. To survive, this doctor learns to keep h/h big mouth shut. If you have such a doctor, the best way to thank h/h is to "husband the resource." Don't try to make h/h talk too much or you'll just dry up this source. Get the information you actually need and no more, then be brief when saying thanks.

◆   ◆   ◆

Crazy, conniving, and insecure types of people add meaningless, distracting drivel when giving for information. This is beyond a waste of time: A doctor asks certain things in certain ways for a reason. Such people may get angry if the doctor tries to steer things back.

In my exam I leave time for things my patient wants to add, but constantly telling me what they want to say instead of answering my questions is not good for them. If a doctor asks, *Do you take any medications?* the answer is *Yes* or *No*, not a two-hour explanation of how you *kind of do*. At best the doctor is concentrating on how to get you back from your side trip quickly without making you angry. It is more likely that you're beginning to confuse h/h focus. Eventually, h/s'll lose attention. That is bad, for you.

If you are unsure of the proper answer don't make a speech starting with, *You really have to hear this, Doc.* Any speech about why the doctor should take the time to let you ramble is poison to the relationship. Doctor's don't take condescension any better than you probably do. Whether you explain their job to them or not, once you say anything like, *You really have to...,* you sound like an obnoxious patient to a doctor's ear.[12]

In summation, in many ways it's better to be the doctor patients are scared to talk to. It's certainly easier and faster. As a doctor there are many things that happen every day that will quiet you down quickly. After enough time these will probably train you to stop bothering to

---

12.   If you can't answer briefly, say you are unsure of what the doctor is asking, and state a brief question about what confuses you.

talk in the first place. For examples of what some of these might be, peek at the next chapter and beyond.

2

Things That Make You Go Hmmmm

Patients legitimately complain of doctors who treat them like a piece of meat. As a doctor, sometimes being elevated to piece of meat from automated slave—droid would be a welcome change. I developed a simple guideline: *I am the most talkative person on earth. If you shut me up you've done something.*

Here are some things doctors deal with all the time. Doctors are bothered by these even if they try not to let it show. Some people do these without realizing it. Some act like the doctor appreciates these things. Wrong. Be sure not to do anything that might even seem like these.

- A doctor asks a question and the patient uses the chance to tell irrelevant stories: Add a star if any involve accusations against other doctors.

- Excessive whining: This turns a doctor into a robot to avoid encouraging it with displays of sympathy. Don't be a drama queen. A doctor can deal with panicky people—that's business as usual. Screaming for attention doesn't make you important. You cannot fool a doctor when it comes to the difference between true panic and a show for attention. In fact, when it comes to reading sympathy acts, doctors are communication geniuses.

- Cars don't chat while being fixed. A doctor is quiet when concentrating. Let h/h be.

- Superstition and religion: Some patients let a doctor know that what h/s does for them is relatively powerless and that the main thing is the magical craft or Voodoo they practice. The doctor becomes wary of talking to them. If your beliefs hinder the way you follow directions let the doctor know in a brief, factual manner so h/s can tell you of the risks. Do not advertise or defend anything, just state the question. This also goes for religious beliefs because one person's religion is the next person's superstition. The treatment can often be modified; if not, tell this to your clergy. Many religions will bend certain rules if your health is at risk.

- Holding the doctor responsible to be perfect: Anything that makes it seem you feel this way (mainly overreacting to human mistakes) is a yellow alert. If a dentist drops something don't go off on how h/s *should be careful, what if that happened in my mouth!* A little joke is okay if it comes off as being understanding, but that's it. Compared with even the greatest athletes, doctors have a fantastic percentage of avoiding human frailty when it counts. Doctors know they are being watched for any sign of imperfection and are scared to so much as drop a pen. Gravity still wins out sooner or later when it comes to such things that don't really matter. As a rule, if you haven't actually been injured by something, ignore it. Beside, why make someone nervous when they could hurt you with a small slip up?

Some doctors don't seem to realize they are being watched. They are sloppy or slovenly and constantly doing things to make you feel that they are probably incompetent, sure to slip up, and not up to medical sanitary standards, to say the least. This becomes your call. Personally, I give a doctor room to be human, but I expect to see h/h wash h/h hands after h/s sneezes into them. If I do something that might appear like it would call for hand cleaning, I'll wash my hands so my patient doesn't have to wonder. If a doctor has you wondering, don't yell at h/h or try to educate h/h. You might say "excuse me, you forgot to scrub…" I might stop using this doctor. If asked why, I would not lie. If everyone did this most of these doctors would get the message. In a setting such as a hospital when you have no freedom to switch doctors (this goes for all staff, not just the doctors and nurses), I might discreetly and politely talk to someone about it. Making a big scene is never the best way to go.

- Taking silence personally: It does not mean you're not interesting. The doctor has little time, so unless you're a movie star or just naturally fascinating, only being medically interesting matters. And remember, to a doctor it's boring unless something is very wrong with you. The ideal is to be the most boring! Put it this way: On *Star Trek* the doctor is often heard to say "My God, I've never seen anything like this before," which increases the interest level. Of course, it is shortly followed by, "He's dead, Jim."

- Focus drifting: It occasionally happens that a doctor does explain well and a patient still doesn't get it. This is rarely because the patient isn't bright enough. It's usually because the patient won't make the effort, has too many preconceptions, or is preoccupied. The preoccupation usually involves thinking up new comments and questions.

Conversation is about the joy of being heard, not the joy of taking in information, except with gossip. We naturally slip into this conversational mode whenever allowed to speak. We spend most of our mental energy preparing our "script" while our doctor drones out h/h lines for the walls to consider.[1] There is no time to teach first grade so a doctor's attitude over time becomes, *do something first to demonstrate a willingness to put mental effort into it.* You are guilty until proven innocent here, but you can have years to win a doctor over

---

1. Reminder: As always, we pay for what all patients do. This doctor may just be tired of patients going through the motions of wanting an explanation when they really want everything done for them. They'd like their insurance to pay for someone to listen to the explanation for them. Asking the questions for them, too, would be nice.

before the real need comes along. Don't wait until crunch time to show you put mental effort into your own health. This is not an option if you are sent to a specialist,[2] but here is a little secret: Don't ask every possible question the first time.[3] Do your homework. If on the second visit it's apparent that your questions are on a higher level or are just to help with your existing studies, doctors become willing discuss things with you. Ask intriguing questions that evidence some deep thought about the information you've taken in and the doctor may become excited to talk with you. Everybody loves to talk about their expertise!

- Resisting the explanation: Some patients habitually, angrily fight for a diagnoses or explanation they want. Nearly everyone will experience a time when h/s tries to influence the diagnoses, probably without realizing it. Be open to the possibility so you can catch yourself.

- Pushing for irrelevant stuff: Allowing the conversation to go this way inevitably leads to some irrelevant limit of the doctor's knowledge that causes many patients to lose confidence. Beside the intrinsically irrelevant academic material, an MD who has worked on nothing but the heart for thirty years may recall little about the eyes. In a "limited" field such as my own, such items as foot disorders don't enter deeply into the equation. If I'd sound lost when a patient brings up toenail fungus, the patient sees me as less of an optometrist. Yet if I say I cannot discuss feet, it's out of my field of expertise, then I might be deemed as being dismissive of the patient's needs.

Now you know of a few "doctor quieting" behaviors. Unfortunately, there are some "doctor quieting" aspects of the relationship that are harder to neutralize. For example, there is the responsibility that

---

2.   Although I know of cases where a doctor knew and respected a patient enough to call ahead and "pave the way" to this kind of relationship, with the specialist.

3.   If there isn't a second visit, the situation is resolved, so who cares. Wise guys/gals are going, "what if that's cause it killed me?" In such an emergency, assuming you were conscious of course, you should have asked.

goes with being given too much credit. If a doctor says, "I like the Chevy," during an exam, some patient would buy one. The professional aura creates a psychological leaning to consider this person as extremely educated no matter the topic. Some people just plain admit to believing everything out of a doctor's mouth.[4] I have even heard apparently rational, intelligent patients say that they accept doctors' opinions on everything in the office because they expect the doctor not to say anything while on the job that isn't on a professional level.

Even though they ignore many of the medical instructions, these very patients act on insignificant nonmedical asides out of a doctor's mouth. The best way to avoid trouble resulting from this canon of doctoral infallibility is to keep quiet. This is especially true about investments because people think doctors know money. Few doctors do. People also believe the doctor gets information from lots of insider clientele and a "doctor network." Patients try to strike up conversations to get investment tips from their doctors. Most doctors steer clear, but some can't resist. They're human—they may be hoping the patient has special information.

So?

There are reasons for doctors to limit communication. This does not change the fact that as a group doctors are poor communicators. The field has developed in ways favoring it, reinforcing selection processes that may favor poor communicators. If for one instant you think most doctors know how to communicate but withhold this from patients, just talk to their support staff; here, as I roughly remember it, is something I saw posted on a bulletin board by a nurses station:

---

4. I have been asked legal questions and found that the person had spoken to a lawyer and wanted me to "overrule" the lawyer, apparently as a greater expert. Well, that seems fair: Bogus medical lawsuits are so easily initiated because attorneys' medical opinions often seem to overrule those of doctors.

Nurses can't understand doctors either

- They don't give clear instructions

- They get high and haughty with us

- Can't understand what they write

- Can't read the handwriting anyway

and patients complain that they also can't understand the nurses!

As far as the tone some doctors take with the nurses, it is probably worse than it ever is with patients. You may be the ignorant client, to some doctors, but nurses are merely hired help. For the vast majority there's the uniquely modern problem of workers not taking orders. You must say "please" very nicely to get someone to do what you pay them to do, and they won't do half of it anyway because it's beneath them. Unfortunately, doctors often need military-type obedience. They need their orders "snapped to." As General Eisenhower discovered when he became president, that stuff don't fly here.

What of the bad handwriting? It is another form of communication trouble and without doubt the legend is based on truth. Many doctors have terrible handwriting, or a great imitation of it on charts and prescriptions. Could there be a connection between the poor communication in conversation and the similar poor communication with pen in hand? The reasons for one might give insight into the other.

So why the bad handwriting?

- Could there be a nuance of, *It's someone else's job to make sense of this, it isn't for me to do it for them by making an effort to write legibly?*

- Maybe they are always too rushed or made to feel that way.

- Is it code? With lawyers looking over their shoulders it might be best to be the only one who knows what is written there. Better yet, even the doctor can't be quite sure.

- Maybe it's left over from the days of the godlike doctors; mere mortals were not meant to comprehend it.

There is no medical course in bad handwriting. People with bad handwritings become doctors. I was told to be a doctor the first time I filled out a registration form in college.

Some people may evolve bad handwritings on purpose because they want what they write to be secret from prying eyes. Perhaps they're naturally born bad communicators: They might have an instinctive sense of keeping things mysterious and making people want to guess at the wisdom they are encoding in their "hieroglyphics." Becoming a doctor, then, fulfils this need to feel like a keeper of mysteries.

My handwriting is world class bad, but consistent in its way, like a code. My charts tend to contain more information than a printout of ten exams by other doctors. I see my handwriting as a "compressed" file. I write too much, too fast. I also speak faster than people can hear if I'm not slowed down once in a while. Do I have a bad handwriting for the opposite reason of other doctors—that I want to say too much? Otherwise, at some point long ago, had these doctors also been kids who wanted to communicate more and faster? If that is the case, what went wrong?

Food for thought indeed. For answers to these and other mysterious questions, be sure to tune in to the next exciting chapter.

3

My Doctor Came From Mercury

What you are about to read has not been corroborated by polling thousands of doctors. It is intended only to give a feel for a doctor's perspective on things.

Doctors are treated like they are from a different planet, and it isn't Venus or Mars. This might make some act as if they are. Doctors are not different. Given their situations most people could understand their behavior and work with them accordingly. It is their situations about which people have complete misconceptions. The experience of giving a medical exam is not at all like the patient being examined might guess. To return the favor doctors somewhat misjudge what it is like to be a patient. Many doctors are shocked by those realities when they become severely ill or take charge of a severely ill relative.

◆   ◆   ◆

Top athletes make tens of millions of dollars per year. This would not be if fans would simply keep their own money for themselves. Too few have ever done so to even show up as statistical blip. At the same time we do many things time to begrudge doctors 1% of that income for saving lives.

Curiously, the real big bucks are made by the few doctors whose income nobody complains about—those who do "luxury" things like cosmetic surgery. They have something in common with athletes and movie stars: They do something nobody needs. Because real medicine is vital, we feel it can't be denied. It's a small leap of logic from there to figuring, *I can keep my money and still expect the care can't be denied.* It's a paradox: The more vital medical care is, the more pressure there is to zero out its value as a service offered on the market. There is no pressure on anyone to provide trivialities, so we accept that we must pay whatever is requested.

We all want the latest mega-expensive drastic technology to be available for us, but we don't want to pay higher premiums because of it. They can raise the premiums if our job pays for it, as long as nobody tells us that this is part of our compensation for working. In other words, don't tell us the increased medical coverage we demanded came in lieu of the raise we expected.

I have been told the seeds of this were evident more than four decades ago, however, it has gone beyond less respect for doctors and begrudging them a nice lifestyle: They are now begrudged a lifestyle that often isn't so nice. Two trends have contributed to this: The schools are churning out too many practitioners and the industry is losing control to huge HMOs and similar employers. Unlike lawyers who thrive under corporate situations that make them seem more necessary than they intrinsically are, doctors are lousy negotiators as a group.

I had a revelation recently. I was in a discussion of the differences between med students and law students with a lawyer of recent vintage and a med school dropout. In my day, when we walked to school uphill both ways in the snow, there was cutthroat competition among pre-med students. In med school the competition was over because a job was waiting for everybody. Pre-law competition wasn't as bad, but in law school the competition for good jobs was fierce.

Well, it seems these days that so many people entered the medical field that there aren't enough jobs. The med-school competition is now killer. I had not known the overabundance of doctors had hit such a level. You can still go into medicine for relative security of nice income, but not for high living. This will make it less likely in the future that the best and the brightest will want to sacrifice so much to be your health care providers and researchers. But at least your software applications will just keep getting better.

As an optometrist I started at the bottom among doctors where I worked. Over the next decade and a half I climbed up because I was willing to deal with management personally, whereas others were scaled down or constantly replaced with somebody making a bit less. It came to the point where some specialties who had been making more than triple my rate were now down to not much more than I had started at—with no adjustment for inflation! In that time my rate had more than doubled. A big help to lowering the wages was switching contract employers twice. At each switch decent salaries were cut or dumped.

People think that even if a hospital is in some ways a big company the management still knows who is a better doctor and reward h/h for it. Actually, things tend to be controlled by larger companies to whom the great doctor is now *employee DX1127*. All that counts is how little h/s'll accept in pay and how many patients h/s'll "process" in a short time. Such systems don't favor more thorough or communicative doctors.

In all situations, including private practice, doctors feel outside forces rushing them; however, insurers, employers, legal agencies, government agencies, suppliers, co-workers, and even many patients give a doctor no credit for doing the same job better by including better communication. H/s is not considered thorough and caring, good, going above and beyond for the same pay, or anything so noble. Just slow and tedious.

If a large corporation has a contract, the people paying them, possibly a state or municipality, have inspectors. If the firm cuts down the number of doctors, they don't care to keep great doctors who work extra hard to give good care to as many patients as possible. Inspectors would see how overworked these doctors are and catch the understaffing. Use a few doctors who adjust by rushing patients through half-hearted exams and by rarely scheduling follow ups, and they will appear to be underworked.

If the corporation doesn't care to keep the better doctors, they will hardly care if they lose the better ones due to lower salaries. Wherever the better ones wind up they are making much less money than they would in a less-corporate-controlled industry.

This is not directly your problem as a patient. I just think you should know about this when I tell you that doctors spend every work day hearing how they make too much money._When it comes to the alleged riches of the average doctor, some people don't recognize where their ignorance lies. An extremely intelligent, open-minded, and generally thorough woman debated this point by saying she saw the bill for individual doctors on a hospital procedure. Just because the bill says ten different care givers (not all doctors) billed separately does not mean anything like that happened.

Insurers, and, especially, government coverage programs, pay less for an overall procedure than they do for its parts, and they may also pay less for an employed doctor than for a self-employed doctor. Employers don't want to make less for this procedure, so they don't bill that way. Instead of hiring care providers they make them partners in a corporation that provides their services back to the real employers. On the bill they are private consultants. They turn the "consultant" proceeds over to the "consulting corporation" that pays h/h a salary. It's all on paper. The money in h/h name goes to the HMO or whatever, and h/s gets a fraction of that kind of income as h/h salary.

There are bigger tricks than this, especially when government coverage is involved. It boils down to a system of, "We pretend to provide reasonable coverage and you pretend to accept this coverage to pay for the service." As long as nobody does things to call public attention to a case, the government and insurers don't want to know.

In the case of facilities billing for allegedly self-employed doctors, the real question is why have different rates for the same service at all: Offer to pay different amounts for the same thing and of course nobody will opt for a lower amount. Even accepting the top amount often involves some compromise. If your car insurance pays too little for repairs, you lose the difference, but the mechanic gets paid. This is not so with direct medical coverage.

Every case is different when it comes to "creative billing." You cannot make a blanket statement about who is cheating whom.

◆   ◆   ◆

The "feel good" concept is that medical care is so important that it can never be denied. It is an ideal condition. It is a good guideline. As an unbendable rule it is the root of many problems. It is the reason many improvements can never be made.

People do take advantage of the idea that care can't be denied. My guess is that 1 or 2% of the patients I see consciously try to take advantage of things, and almost all of us eventually do something without realizing that it results from having thought along these lines. In the middle are people who spend money on less important things without a thought to planning for "a rainy day," and eventually barter/plead/ scream for a break on their health care.

Ultimately, doctors must provide. Negotiating the price of a service you can't withhold is like negotiating a price for your watch with an armed robber.

For all those wondering if socialized medicine is the answer, it is if you don't like good health care. It provides little profit to support research and development. All the "Western" countries providing it keep it afloat on some hidden supports, such as:

- If I get really sick and have money I'll pay for better treatment, maybe in the USA.

- Med labs around the world exist to sell in the USA. American prices get extra high to make up for lack of profit elsewhere. Countries with socialized medicine tend to buy minimal amounts of each new technology. They can claim to provide it, but you might be on a waiting list for years. Hence, people come here for (immediate) treatment. Once the technology has cheapened, it goes everywhere cheap—thank you, USA, for paying the real bill. Socialized medicine would have fallen apart everywhere had we gone with it!

◆   ◆   ◆

A doctor is very aware that the real world is full of lawyers. Let's say someone requests bifocals, but I believe it would be too much for h/h to get used to presently. No matter what guarantees h/s gives, when h/s trips for a completely unrelated reason some lawyer will take the case. The fact that I gave warning only serves to prove that I was aware of a danger and didn't save this person from h/hself.

The doctor has this dilemma: The patient must be given the chance to make certain decisions but if they aren't happy with the results of that decision the fault is still, ultimately, the doctor's. Most people in the doctor's position might find some way around getting into this conundrum in the first place. That might involve saying as little as possible so patients can't even guess at the options there are.

◆   ◆   ◆

Many doctors actually do not think they are god, but some patients act like doctors are above human feelings and can make up for all patient transgressions cheerfully. Very few will say, "You are a bad patient, leave;" however, doctors don't actually think, *I must treat everyone nice no matter what.* Some may think, *It's easiest if I appear to treat everyone nice no matter what.* If a patient thinks h/s pulled one over on the doctor, it's because the doctor wants h/h to think that. This makes h/h all the easier to handle. Although that great *Seinfeld* episode exaggerated (a lot) about what happens next, doctors do take defensive measures (such as giving out impossible appointment times) and may warn friends about the worst patients.

This is especially true when a doctor medically has no choice but to refer a bad patient to a specialist. I want a specialist to appreciate my referrals. I do not want all of my patients to suffer because a couple of bad patients made the specialist wary of me. The specialist might wonder if I am a bottom feeder with only bad patients, or if I simply dump my worst ones on h/h.

You might wonder how that can be—the specialist must see that there was a medical reason for each referral! Not necessarily. That's only for patients referred because I know they have a serious condition. Some are referred because I require the specialist's opinion to determine that. Some things that look potentially scary to a general practitioner are seen instantly as harmless by the specialist. The specialist could wonder if I was quick to put the diagnosing in h/h hands with the unpleasant patients—for all h/s knows I send nice patients with real problems elsewhere!

Here is a great example of dumping a bad kind of patient that worked out for everyone. I knew a dentist with certain specialties. He also had a medical condition himself. He had no sense of smell. Some perfectly nice patients have bad breath. Some simply do not have the courtesy to brush their teeth for a year or so before coming. All the lucky dentists anywhere near this guy simply found excuses to refer "foul mouthed" patients to him. He then handled all of their dental needs. For those with genuine conditions causing the odor, he truly was their specialist: He probably knows more about it due to seeing more of these people than any other dentist. Despite being the expert on causes of halitosis, however, he probably was not good at diagnosing it: He'd always be the last to know if someone had bad breath.

◆   ◆   ◆

Let's concede that it is best to treat a patient as a person rather than a set of symptoms. We then accept that a doctor should get a good case history at the start and should explain what the story is at the end. In between it's still better to do tests objectively, as if the patient is a machine. Patient personality must be considered for the talking at the start and the end, but neutralized for the testing in the middle. Some doctors just eliminate it from the equation altogether since their training may be over 95% for the middle part. Some just eliminate it because it's easier. The thing is, I find the remaining 4 or 5 % might be the most important.

Some doctors are personality geniuses who intuitively take into account what a therapist would take years to uncover. Even so, some of these doctors don't act in a "human" way: It is easier to use personality facts as such, facts. For doctors without this gift there is some safety in acting robotically.

It actually would be more accurate to say that during the middle 95% it is the doctor who treats h/hself as a machine in trying to eliminate h/h own personality from affecting the results. The patient is still going to affect the tests with h/h personality. To get the objective results as if the patient was a car's transmission, a doctor really has to be constantly aware that there is a person down there who has a personality that is hampering the objectivity and account for that! Treating you like a machine can be a way of trying to get you to neutralize your own clouding of the accuracy. Unfortunately, it is also sometimes just a bad doctor treating you like a machine. It also can backfire if a patient reacts to such treatment.

To assist doctors who may act this way for good reason, patients should observe doctors. Work to get a sense of who is trying to keep you logical (machinelike) in your responses at critical times and who is just a robot h/hself when it comes to the interpersonal stuff.[1] Don't take offense at either. Doctors may not realize they do this or how it comes out in the patient's view. Doctors should try being patients without letting it be known that they are doctors. Observe for these same behaviors, then watch yourselves closely when you are back at work.

Patients should try to be "coldly" objective in responses when it seems the doctor is asking for that—one reason doctors make bad patients is that they know too much and they can't keep that from affecting the answers. As for the "cold fish" doctor, if h/s is otherwise a great doctor, deal with it the best you can. If you can't deal with it anymore, or if h/s isn't worth it, find a doctor you can work with more smoothly. Don't try to change this doctor. It can't work.

Some people like a doctor who is a robot who treats them like a robot. They are embarrassed by being examined and by the treatments, and prefer it to be done as coldly and distantly as possible! Some in the field of psychology who tell us all this stuff make a point of advertising how cold and distant they will be while listening to all that their patient's have to say.

If a doctor's personality is truly unbearable by most people's opinions, then h/s will find it hard to keep enough patients. If that doctor is so great that h/s still gets patients, then h/s has the right to offer h/h skill and personality as a package deal and everyone can accept it or choose a better personality with lesser skills.

◆   ◆   ◆

There are powers a doctor doesn't control to which h/s may even answer. H/s may be employed by or accept payment from bureaucratic-style organizations. Insurers and union and government agencies mess up. Low-level individuals working there like power. A person in

---

1.   No offense to *Star Trek's* "Data" and other such artificial life forms who put in the superhuman effort to communicate on deep and sympathetic levels.

such a position can say "yes" or "no." "Yes" is what everyone wants. Say it, people say "thanks," and are done with you. Say "no" and they need to beg, scream, plead, bargain, threaten, argue, etc., etc. They are in h/h sphere of command and must stay there. These mini-Napoleons crave small tastes of power and they only get it by saying, "NO!"

Patients rarely come face to face with these people. It's always phone calls, letters, email, forms, or asking someone else (such as a union rep, or an insurance agent, or the doctor's staff) to ask for you. People need someone to blame who is there to hear it. Well, the doctor is there, and h/s must ultimately be in charge; after all, h/s's the doctor! Doctors take lots of blatant and subtle abuse due to shortcomings of the patient's coverage or the hospital's systems.

Complaints with bureaucracies often involve treatments the patient wants but can't get. This becomes more common when third parties are paying. When patients pay they usually go the other way: They see conspiracies whenever they're told they need anything. Sometimes they'll mention that they can't afford it and the doctor says that h/s will do the minimum anyway because it's vital. Some will suddenly agree that they need the treatment and in fact the doctor is cheating them out of the rest which obviously is also vital and should be included, free.

Although some doctors do extra things to pad the bill,[2] many accusations come from the "imaginations" of patients, especially from those who are angling for something. Thousands of doctors who have never cheated by a penny hear these accusations outright or as asides every day. A "wink wink nudge nudge" comment to this effect is not a diplomatic way to open the channels of communication. Such a person does not seem like someone who is "in" on the setup and is willing to be cool with it—h/s seems like a jerk to be avoided.

---

2.   There are many legitimate reasons a doctor will do something that may not be medically necessary; for example, protection from lawsuits. There's also the human quirk of seeing everything as needing our particular help.

It is possible to run into a doctor who is manipulating for more profit by extra treatment. If you believe you have fallen into the care of such a doctor, switch doctors. More often than not you will never be sure and might never be able to do anything about it anyway. It doesn't matter whether the doctor really is pulling anything. You are not comfortable. The problem, therefore, isn't what the doctor does; it's your choice to stay with a doctor who makes you uncomfortable. Switch. Otherwise, the problem is now your fault, so stop bothering people about it.

If you actually have proof of misdoings, take it to the authorities. That is no longer a medical matter, but a legal one. Don't hang around looking for more dirt because you are consumed with vengeance. Don't stay with this crook because you believe you now have leverage. All of these are reasons to get two new doctors: One to replace this fellow for your health care, and another one for your obvious mental health dysfunctions.

◆   ◆   ◆

As we've discussed, doctors feel they are held to standards of perfection. Doctors eventually learn to bristle at the slightest intimation of any human imperfection. You know what can lead to human mistakes and lots of other things? Monotony. A doctor's work is important, it's not necessarily interesting or special. If a person is really bored, they may not even want to discuss the topic that bores them. Your doctor may be thinking of last night's game when you come in. Believe it or not, it's a job, maybe for much longer than 8 hours strait. Don't believe that just because serious things happen that makes it any different.

Medicine is less like TV than any other "exciting life" profession, and they're all boring. Lawyers, cops, etc., spend most of the time doing dull, repetitive stuff, followed by paperwork and time when nothing is happening. The few things that would be exciting to us become boring to them. Things have to become boring to be surviv-able. If we lived in a foxhole we'd normalize that because nobody can survive being on adrenaline 24 hours a day. Soldiers tell stories of men getting wounded or killed because they eventually just get careless under nonstop fire.

We want a doctor who's cool and calm, qualities that come from familiarity with the situation, which means boredom, which means a doctor's mind can wander. If things were so exciting to h/h that h/h mind couldn't lose focus, you would probably be in big trouble. Either h/s is someone who is constantly overwhelmed, or it must be your situ-ation that is overwhelming. The moment h/s acknowledges that by becoming excited, h/s's dropped at least a notch in h/h ability to help.

I know right away what is the general case with about 90% of patients who enter my exam room. The rest is details, formalities, and unrelated screenings. The routine is all very routine, unless your prob-lem is far from routine. So, pretty much unless you have a new breed of alien crawling out of your body, the doctor might be bored, or at least working on autopilot.

Lucy, you got some 'splainin to do.

Explaining is an art. Some doctors find it hard to explain things to patients. Some find it hard to explain anything in general. They were tested in med school for understanding (actually, for repetition of facts), not for how they can explain it to someone else. In orals they may be tested for accuracy when explaining it to someone who knows it better than they do. They are not tested for whether someone could actually learn anything from their explanations.

My grandfather would use a saying: *If you can't explain it you don't really understand it.* That depends on what level of understanding is required. Some people do have enough functional understanding to operate (loaded choice of words), but not enough theoretical compre-hension to explain. Even if you do, there's no time to teach from the ground up. Most people have nearly zero basic science understanding or, worse, lots of wrong "knowledge."

There's an art to taking a complicated thing requiring years of study and providing a feel for the concept in minutes. Most doctors simply shake their head *yes* to many popular misconceptions because it's the easiest way to have you think you understand.

There's also a "playing telephone" element. No matter how painstakingly I explain and make sure every piece is understood properly, it comes back later incredibly wrong. It's safer to say nothing than to have someone insist you said something that you didn't come close to saying. Some people are so certain they'll be confused they guarantee it. Simple sentences get reactions as if they were all of quantum mechanics rolled into one sentence.

◆   ◆   ◆

Your doctor faces this quandary: H/s has to get you to be serious about not missing an appointment or a referral or the taking of a pill, yet h/s must not scare you too much. Patients get so scared they figure it's pointless, or they panic or even go into denial.[3] It is hard to know just how to reduce things, to what degree...

This patient now requires a super message while being a lousy receiver. This must be an interaction even though the patient may say nothing. It takes a special sense to tell how much the receiver is understanding, how to modify your words or what to emphasize, what must be repeated and what would insult their intelligence by being repeated, what they must be told and what they can't deal with, how their expectations or ulterior motives affect how they take things in, and where's the fine line between enough to make them serious and committed and

---

3.   Some doctors go the other way and have an element of doctor as coach: "Use pills this way" comes with a pep talk. Unfortunately, pep talks by nature stray from the truth.

so much it scares them into panic, denial, or anger. This sounds very similar to the sense I discussed as being truly the *sense* of humor.

Beyond using this sense, humor by its nature is the most flexible communication medium to give as much info as each receiver can deal with; however, the sense must be highly attuned because used incorrectly the presence of humor will be considered offensive. It is still a tool. Knifing a patient would be offensive, too, but that doesn't mean a scalpel has no use in medicine. It just means it should be used with surgical precision so it doesn't seem to be a dagger.

How many people can communicate smoothly on such a level? Without special training? Whatever combination of innate talent, training, and practice is required, few people have it; and no real training is given. Most people, therefore, would say the minimum necessary to be able to claim they said what had to be said. Beside, this is all very stressful, so there's a nervous urge to be out of there. Add to this the fact that any extra word could be the one to start trouble and most people would just mumble something and move on. Sound like any kind of person you know?

◆   ◆   ◆

Doctors are uneasy with any words put into their mouths. Here are a few guidelines.

- If you want to diagnose yourself, leave the doctor out of it

- The doctor can't prescribe what you have decided to get

- The doctor can't debunk an infinite amount of things you read into h/h words

- A purely imaginary thing often can't be debunked. If you insist there are purple subatomic mice-men telepathically controlling your arm hair, well there you have it, I guess. Now, it sounds crazy, which is why people steer things to: *So what you're saying, Doc, basically, is that you think I have purple subatomic...*

Once you seem to have put words into a doctor's mouth, h/s probably figures the more h/s says, the more you'll misquote. Misquotes do make it to courts of law. Even when it is admitted that the doctor said it correctly and wrote it correctly and triple checked that the patient understood, the doctor is still nervous that h/s'll be held accountable for the patient's later distortion of the information.

The more a doctor says, the more likely h/s'll actually make a mistake. Even if h/s catches and corrects it, in some ways it can never be stricken from the record. Some people forget which was the thing they were told to "strike from the record, it's a mistake."

Now it gets even more convoluted. Doctors disagree. People accept this intellectually. However, when this comes up in the real world people can't deal with this reality. Doctors constantly deal with patients who talk about the differences of another doctor's methods. There is obviously some reason they no longer see this doctor, but in the new doctor's office the other one might as well have been god.

Emotionally, people want absolutes from their doctors. They need it to be medical science. Science is the working realm of researchers. Practitioners work in the medical arts.

Doctors who may respect each other's methods still don't want their patients discussing treatments with enough detail to see that there's a difference. The more that is explained, the more likely this becomes. It can be as simple as some doctors attack with every medicine right away, yet others prefer using as little medicine as possible. Neither is absolutely right or wrong. The special doctor doesn't have some magic right answer. What makes h/h special is the sense of when and how a treatment needs adjusting or altering. When nothing available works, greatness may be seen in improvising.

Greatness is dangerous. Say a genius knows the standard treatment is risky in your case compared with something h/s has been devising. Results of this new method will not be compared with what would have been on average; it will be compared with perfection. The last thing a doctor with the guts to help this way needs is to supply the patient with enough information to start headaches for the doctor.

Now things are just starting to heat up. What if the condition itself is one of those mystery ailments, like lower back pain. Lots of people have it. Big pain can mean big problems, little problems, or even problems with no discernable physical basis. To a degree this applies to any pain anywhere, but the difficulty in finding the cause for many real lower backaches (and headaches) makes them very popular complaints for people who feel no pain. Especially after minor or alleged accidents. Nobody can ever absolutely prove they are lying.

Doctors do not want to start up with people who are faking. Even when it's obvious doctors can only be hurt, sometimes physically, by doing anything about it. If a person doesn't make it too obvious that nothing is wrong or if the person believes it h/hself the doctor has a tendency to see things that way too. It is human nature. A doctor does not like to feel that something is beyond h/h control or outside h/h jurisdiction.

There is a saying; *If you give a monkey a hammer everything is a nail.* Any person, no matter how brilliant or simple minded, can be that monkey. People see everything as needing their help and the tools of their trade. Take a car accident. Cops see it as primarily a law enforcement situation and that their emergency authority is the most important. Medical people see it first and foremost as a medical emergency. A fireman might think that preventing a major explosion is key and should override other considerations. Of course, some lawyer ultimately takes charge and to "mark h/h turf" h/s will check on how everyone who actually handled the crisis performed.

The monkey—hammer concept tells us that each specialist sees an ailment as needing h/h touch. It leads to friction between similar or overlapping specialties. It also means it needs the latest hammer at h/h disposal. Provide ultraexpensive, superadvanced equipment and it must be used: Everything must be fixable by it. It will eventually become thought of as standard. At that point it must always be used just in case something unrelated goes wrong because some lawyer will have it on a list of mandatory routine tests. Long before this point the doctor tends to see things in terms of, *Boy, are you lucky this happened today, a month ago we didn't have this technology to irradiate that hangnail.*

This becomes one of our examples of what appears to be overdoing things to bill for more exotic procedures, but is really just a normal human reaction to getting that hammer. It is best to realize this before questioning the need for a procedure: Don't make it an accusation, you will not get you what you want. Try asking, "How would you have handled this a week before they invented that machine?"

To tie it all together, people with mysterious ailments and doctors with the newest, biggest hammers are an interesting mix.

As I was finishing this chapter I had an experience that is an excellent example of the complexity of the communication task for a doctor.

A patient honestly answered that he had no medical condition. He has been diabetic for so long it is the normal state to him. He only thinks of it as something to discuss as a medical condition when it gets out of control. This is not unusual. When I discovered he was diabetic I instructed him to remember to report that to any doctor who asks in the future.

I often start the explaining process that prior physicians and nurses left for later. I suspect there's an element of, *I'm just diagnosing, explaining is for the long-term doctors,* later followed by, *the doctor who diagnosed this must have done the necessary explaining.* I've seen this happen even when the same doctor or team both diagnosed and did the long-term care, as long as they didn't know from the start that they would be doing it all.

Patients compound this problem. They don't want bad news so they don't ask questions that could lead to bad news. Then they convince themselves that if it was bad they'd have been told. The patient eventually may realize there were questions to be asked, but after all this time of acting as if h/s knew enough h/s doesn't want to seem stupid.

Okay, so I actually talked to this patient who was told of his diabetes years earlier. Because it never came up before this was apparently the first time he thought about it. His question came out so innocently he didn't even realize enough to feel ignorant. He asked, *Is this diabetes in any way a bad thing? At all? Should I have any little concerns? Should I consider any form of treatment?*

Be honest, if you were in a bar and someone said the word diabetes and a discussion ensued would it occur to you to say to the guys (and gals), *By the way, diabetes is a bad thing to have. It is actually preferable not to have it.*

So, if an intelligent adult asks you what you know of diabetes, do you talk to h/h like a three year old? Should you assume h/s has a college education with emphasis on the sciences and start at a high level? Somewhere in between? Will the person actively and wisely guide the levels and fine tuning of your answers? Would a person be embarrassed to say h/s needs the three-year-old level? Would the same person see it as condescending if you started by explaining the most basic levels? It's difficult, even for a great speaker, and that's not Dr Johnny.

The same dilemma is faced by the patient when saying things to the doctor. I have observed miscommunications with other kinds of experts that provided some insights. There was a time I had my brakes checked and was told that nothing was wrong. I knew something was wrong, but I was told again and again that there was no problem. I eventually deduced that the mechanics were being too literal in looking for a brake problem when I said there was a problem with my brakes. I changed my complaint to "a problem when braking."

I was dealing with a variation of the professor who can't relate to what students don't understand. These experts would never think brakes when it's a master cylinder problem. They forgot that to the layman stopping system problems are braking problems. I asked to have the brakes checked and literally, the brakes were checked, not every related system.

Doctors must learn to translate the generalizations of laymen. Patients should remove any level of diagnosis from the statement of a complaint. If moving your arm a certain way causes a pain in your shoulder, say, *My shoulder feels a sharp pain here when I move my arm this way.* Don't say, *Check my shoulder, there's something wrong with it.* The problem may not be in the shoulder. It is amazing how long it can take the doctor, patient, specialists, nurses, and anyone else, to realize nothing is being found because everybody jumped on an innocent misdirection.

We have accepted that doctors are not great communicators and now we also see that there are reasons a doctor isn't motivated to talk very much or very well. I find it amazing the way people spend hundreds of dollars per hour to talk to a lawyer to complain that their doctor won't talk limitlessly for free…And these patients aren't always world class communicators themselves. There are even patients who come in with motivations beside getting good and efficient health care. Knowing what they are like is important.

It does not matter how few of them there are. It does not matter that you are not one of them. They affect how the doctor acts at all times, more than even h/s may realize. If you seem like them for even a moment your task becomes much more difficult. To get around the obstacles to good communication with a doctor you should know a little about them so…

Stay tuned for next thrilling chapter to see…

The thing that invaded my office

4

Why do bad people happen to good things?

This chapter is an attempt to give about 98% of patients a feel for what the others are like. With luck it will help some doctors: We can only control our behavior patterns by accepting that we are molded by patient interactions. It can only help to have some specific types of interactions pointed out.

Whatever your doctor is up against, you, as the good patient trying to communicate, are also up against! The communication challenge involves the doctor's and the patient's personalities and situations. The doctor's situation involves (and h/h personality reflects) the personalities of all of h/h patients, ever. Real experience has molded h/h behavior despite all idealism. The self-preservation instinct is involved, h/s doesn't keep doing what caused h/h pain before. To paraphrase the safe sex warning, *You are not just having a communication problem with h/h, you are having a communication problem with every patient h/s has ever had contact with.*

I often mention that patients will sue. Far more often they become personally abusive, complain, write letters, spread rumors, and cause various annoyances without suing. I tend to sum it up with the dramatic, "the patient may sue," because the only time most doctors (and good patients) seem to consider the whole dynamic is to talk of the big problem, the suit. Even a doctor who has not been sued pays obscene malpractice insurance rates due to the probability it will happen. Guess who ultimately foots that bill, good patient.

I've previously alluded to an episode of *Seinfeld* about "The List." *Elaine* glanced over her own chart and wanted a note changed. A new note went in and no doctor would ever give her the time of day after that. It isn't quite as simple as that, but doctors do remember when someone has been abusive. Doctors put things in the record when it can be a legal matter; for instance, when a patient violently argues against the doctor's proper recommendation. When the patient's self-fulfilling prophecy that medical care won't help h/h plays out, the doctor must have it in the record. Being concerned with communication as we are, the mythological list is irrelevant. The list of problem patients in your doctor's head and charts, or known to his staff, matters.

Some people freely show the worst side of themselves in a doctor's office, similar to when "alcohol does their speaking," free of normal inhibitions. It may be because patients have to open up to tell of embarrassing problems, or get undressed and be poked and prodded. What Elaine did was nothing compared with what doctors put up with every day. The implication that doctors put up with very little was a source of comedy in that *Seinfeld*. Real doctors put up with incredible abuse before they even notice, and then many still put up with it because they have no idea how to deal with it "professionally". They don't jump on minor transgressions, but they do anticipate and are defensive over horrific ones.

Generations ago the truly obnoxious patients may have been a once-a-year oddity. They are still a tiny percentage, but they no longer qualify as rare. More than one is seen by any doctor per week, if not per day. I knew of a third-generation doctor who, circa the late 1970s, refused to let his kids become doctors. He wasn't going to let them be abused that way!

◆   ◆   ◆

Some people like to make others miserable for the sheer joy of it, but for most people being annoying is not an end in itself. We all know some born nuisances, but they probably don't plan how they can bother people. Doctors face some people who are nuisances on purpose, basically for profit. Profit can be many things, such as getting freebies, extra time and attention, or a discount on the bill. The ultimate scam is always aimed at a *settlement*, and that comes from a lawsuit, or to avoid a lawsuit.

Lawsuits are easy to understand, here are a couple examples of less obvious but more common nuisance *for profit* activities. Some are done on purpose, others are behavior patterns that have simply "evolved" over time because they have been "rewarded."

- Lonely people use the idea that if they claim something is wrong the doctor must spend time with them. A huge amount of complaints are made about good glasses because optometrists rarely charge when complicated cases need extra visits. Lonely people with good coverage spend quality time with their physician in search of mystery ailments. In institutional settings complaints can easily become accusations.

- Some people hope to squeeze out something for free by complaining. In my field most offices just give them what they want to maintain good relations. It doesn't work. You simply train them to come back and try for even more in the future.

◆   ◆   ◆

Certain people take offense at everything. If you say they left out their date of birth they shout, *Why you spying on my age*! Let's say the record has an "unlikely" bit of information that is relevant to the diagnosis. It may not be a typo, the patient may have "helped" the mistake get into the record. Some lie to get the doctor to skip the test for whatever they know or fear they have. Some figure if they fudge things like the family history they'll get a better report, which makes them feel good. They then cement their denial by reasoning that their lies couldn't have fooled a professional, so the results are accurate.

Some patients are convinced the doctor is using info to trick them. They'll manipulate answers to prevent this. They might reveal things at the end like, *Oh yeah, I do take medications, here they are, what do you think now? I started them after my stroke—which I also didn't tell you about.*

Patients who distort information and testing are tolerated due to the premise that doctors must always help and act professionally. I advocate a subpremise of "tough professionalism." Quietly letting patients misbehave should not be confused with professional demeanor. If politeness interferes with information, testing, instructions, or the welfare of the patient in any way, then don't be nice.

Doctors definitely have this ability. Earlier in my career I had trouble doing certain tests because I was too nice to the patients. In my profession we do relatively few of these things compared with doctors who poke, prod, cut and drill all the time. They know how to *just do it*; for instance, when popping your shoulder back into its socket. Many otherwise excellent doctor candidates can't overcome the urge to be kind and gentle when a sharp tug is called for. Every graduate managed to! Few translate this ability into their speech.

I have progressed so far that when a patient won't sit still, assuming the test is vital, I go beyond getting physically determined and become verbally tough. It works. When I first did it I braced for complaints: There were only apologies for how hard they made it for me. People don't react to what actually happened; they react the way that you show them you'll allow. One's manner may wear a "kick me" sign, or a "grovel before me" sign, or anything in between. It reads, and so shall ye be treated.

◆   ◆   ◆

There are patients who halt the exam for long-winded talks. The doctor must steer things back to business. There's a type who get very angry at this. They'll explain why they must re-re-explain and may add a hollering, berating "lesson." They'll interrupt to say how rude the doctor is. All the while, they're making it impossible to put together any information that counts. Anything that matters will be stated several contradictory ways, all of which may be wrong and all of which are later denied.

To moderate such things a doctor may indeed do what would be a rude in another setting, but it is as improper to label this as rude as it would be for a student to call a teacher rude for running a class. Lecturers, standup comedians, teachers, parents, employers, generals, judges, and many others have certain permitted modes of discourse that are not coequal conversation. So do doctors. To be rude one must do something outside of one's permitted mode.[1]

I accept the games of the worst patients as a small price for encouraging communication, and in fact I see it as a chance to observe some fascinating behaviors up close. I can, however, certainly understand how another doctor might come to avert these uncomfortable hours of wasted time by avoiding all conversation. As an added bonus this way h/s can never be accused of having rudely stopped any specific statement!

◆   ◆   ◆

Our concept of co-equality becomes misused. Your doctor may pay lip service to whatever concept h/s has found brings h/h the least grief, ignore what any doctor says on this count: You should know how to

---

1.   I am never rude. I raise obnoxiousness to artistic levels, but politely.

sidestep this *relationship minefield* whether your doctor knows h/s reacts to this or not.

The doctor and you are partners in your health care, our "psychoba-bblephilic" society insists on saying equals. Risking the wrath of the Political Correctness Industrial Complex, such semantics can be dangerous. Instead of making people realize they have responsibility to work with their doctor for their health, these words are used to block the doctor from discussing the patient's lack of taking responsibility. *How dare you tell me that—I'm co-equal you know!*

Responsible patients ask what more they can do. I have heard patients who felt a doctor was condescending say something like, *I am not an idiot, and since taking care of myself is up to me I would appreciate it if you would tell me what I need to know.* They don't babble about equality. If you want respect for your intelligence, show some. If the doctor gives a pep talk mentioning your equal status, fine. Don't just sit there feeling warm and fuzzy about it: It's not about accomplishments, it's about your responsibility ahead.

It's funny, it suddenly isn't co-equal when things go wrong. Your health is your main job; to a doctor it's one of countless lives h/s's divided between helping. Because doctors don't sue patients, courts only deal with the doctor's responsibility. Anytime courts get involved letting only one side profit from being a victim, people on that side will make themselves victims. That's why pedestrians look down and walk right in front of moving cars. Some of these cars are driven by people who will in turn sue GM or Ford over brakes that were 50,000 miles overdue for maintenance. Considering how patient irresponsibility can transmit diseases or even create things like antibiotic-resistant microbes, it may be time for courts to put some onus on the recipients of medical technologies.

The doctor is an expert you employ to assist in your responsibility. You have one power: Fire h/h. Between the hiring and firing h/s is the expert. Respect your own decision to pick this doctor.

The co-equality concept makes people feel like talk time should be equal. Big mistake. We want information. We should not be there for conversation or to fuel our egos. Ask a question then take notes like a student in class. If you don't act like the one getting information, then trust me, you won't. Fighting for equal time can be insulting, we are being dismissive of h/h expertise and time constraints in order to babble. A doctor is our teacher dissertating, not our friend discussing.

To summarize, the phrase co-equals and all similar things used to lower the doctor a peg or two is like a scalpel. A doctor may use it; a patient picking it up is threatening. You, the patient, have the main responsibility. The doctor has more authority. Responsibility and authority are apples and oranges, so equal is an illogical concept.

People with terrible self-images play a game of "we're equal, don't think you're better." It isn't a matter of being treated decently: In no individual moment can anyone seem better than them. I have witnessed such people insulting the heroes trying to save their relative during emergency procedures. If their interference bungles the attempt, they use the failure as proof to back their insults. Then, of course, comes "blame and sue." The worse they are, the greater their need for denial and blaming, the more viciously they lash out.

◆   ◆   ◆

We've touched on how self-paying patients question anything for which they'll have to pay, whereas patients covered by third parties question anything they don't get. Self-payers opt for less expense, so the covered patient is often getting more service. Nevertheless, doctors constantly hear how much more some covered patients think they should get, or their demands to get "what the *others* get." You are just more likable to anybody if you show some appreciation for what you are getting.

As a patient, if I believe there is something I could use that is not covered, I have the same option to pay for it as a self-paying patient. I would save any discussion of what should be covered for my insurance agent. H/s would let me know how much more expensive such a policy would be.

In my experience, the more distant the person from the payment, the greater the complaint. Self-payers may mention price, but not service. People who pay their own premiums have a sense of having chosen an expense vs. coverage compromise. People who get coverage through an employer have a tendency to compare things with some magical billion-dollar policy. If the government, or some charity, is footing the bill, some people demand the magical, billion-dollar treatment.

Saying, *The Government doesn't pay enough,* might as well be saying, *The doctor doesn't do enough.* When the patient complains to the doctor that the government should also pay for other add ons, the message is that something should be done about it. Because the only person who can hear this attack is the doctor, it's easy to see at whom this message of "somebody should do more for me" is aimed. Considering that the doctor may be compensated less than h/h costs so this work is basically charity, you can guess how enthusiastically these complaints are received.

This is not a matter of political philosophy. A doctor might be a political activist for such government programs, but if that very doctor hears how h/s is somehow ripping off the person h/s is helping, h/s doesn't learn to like this person.

◆   ◆   ◆

Some people hold their own health hostage to control the doctor. People extend the, *Why pay, why save for this emergency since a doctor must help me anyway,* behavior to, *Why show up on time or make any effort at all.* [2] Without anyone consciously putting it into words, the

---

2.   Like the bad drivers who put on those "baby on board" signs then drove even worse because it was now your responsibility to care for their baby's welfare.

evolved behavior is taught by example down the generations. Patients have literally bargained with their health, some have said to me that they will follow my instructions if I do something *in return* for them! Because one's health is ultimately the doctor's problem to such a patient, h/s will catch a doctor on h/h off time for free consultations. No matter how rudely the patient acts to set up this "chance" [3] conversation the doctor is now cast as rude and unprofessional. This is as opposed to lawyer who might bill you for a chat at a party.

It's called the waiting room for a reason

If any complaint is more universal than the way doctors communicate, it's the one about waiting times. We want thorough exams, increased communication, personal attention, when we feel we need to be seen even on short notice, and with an exact start time—but we may be late.

A truly short wait will not happen until we are willing to pay so much that all doctors allot slots like psychiatrists and only see about eight patients a day, who pay even if they miss their exam. The rates we pay are based on the doctor seeing scores of patients.

How many of us make it our business to do everything possible to get in promptly and get through it quickly? You can't have an efficient medical office unless the single biggest factor is efficient. That factor is not the doctor, nurses, office staff, or any equipment. It's the patients.

Some people are talented at stealing time. They ask a doctor to stay late or to squeeze them in because they came late. They'll walk in unscheduled and act as if the staff's at fault: "But I already made the trip[4], so 'schedule' me for now!" They'll often lie about an emergency

---

3. Many of the behaviors discussed in this book have come to my attention directly from the parties behaving this way. They tell stories of their obnoxious behavior and complain about the reactions of the doctors, nurses, staff workers, or fellow patients. They have no clue that anything they ever do is ever seen as improper. To them rudeness, unfairness, abusiveness, and the like are all like gravity, only applying toward themselves.

4. This is oft times untrue: They drop in when they are nearby for other reasons.

nature of the problem, yet add that it's nothing that will take a lot of time. Once in the exam room they start advising the doctor, *There's no need to rush, you shouldn't rush this, this is important.*

Patients who cause the need to rush are aware to watch for it. If they make accusations, the very fact that they caused the rush is proof that there was a rush! The doctor feels h/s must prove h/s is not rushing so they may get more than normal time. These are never emergencies: True "urgencies" need no conniving to get in, and an actual emergency is generally in an ambulance bound for an emergency room. You don't have to wonder how time-stealing patients might somehow affect your interaction with the doctor. They are the reason you have to wait so long for so little interaction time.

A communication cure to this would be for the doctors to say, *You swore you needed so little time you can be squeezed in, now you've changed your mind. We cannot take that much time from other patients. No problem, go schedule an actual exam and since this was never intended to be one we'll only charge a "consultation" fee for today. Because those are not covered arrange payment on your way out.* They could comply, or switch doctors. Unfortunately, they won't switch. They will beg for a quick look and swear that's all they ever said it required. I know this to be true—I put my theories through real-world tests.

I once worked in a building with a shared waiting room where my office door was the only one that opened directly to the waiting room. When I'd catch patients squeezing their names into the middle of my sign-in sheet I'd move them. These people were generally unprepared for anyone standing up to them, but some tried to push their luck. On more than one occasion I received actual applause from the waiting room "audience." I am therefore certain that most patients want the abusive patients set straight.

Some doctors are too swamped to realize what's going on when the staff squeezes in patients. If a doctor is always overloaded and doesn't seem to care, I'd avoid h/h. If a doctor doesn't resent having the schedule squeezed, h/s could be one of those doctors who want all the "business" possible and the assembly line of "care" can't move fast enough.

Crowding can also be due to how special a doctor is. I subtract points for rushed care and long waits before deciding whether anyone's special enough. As Yogi Berra would say, "Nobody goes there anymore, it's too crowded."

◆   ◆   ◆

There are patients who ask for detail far beyond any reasonable need. The doctor may be damned if h/s doesn't answer and damned worse if h/s does. Provide an in-depth answer and the effort the patient must sustain gets one type agitated, even it's just the effort to appear to make an effort. They try rephrasing their questions, making less and less sense until it's just static. They become frustrated and angry. They really want to feel they've done a great job and that they must seem like a special patient to the doctor. When you surprise them with what they asked for, they are confused by how little they want it.

The solution would be to give them great compliments for asking and an excuse why we can't go that deeply into things now. That's fine for the second time around, once we know what type they are. The only way to tell this, unfortunately, is by answering the first time.

There are also those who manage to go straight to anger from the start of any explanation. They probably just want control. They put out questions to get a feel for ordering the doctor to do something: *Answer. Dance. Quack like a duck.* Making them listen to answers is rebellious against their control, and it ruins their negotiating position. They assume you won't answer, but that you'd grant something in exchange.

I can gauge what they are after by how angry they get while I answer. Some ultimately want things they are not entitled to medically, or at least not through their coverage. They've sometimes wanted illegal things. Rage is defensive: When having their motives revealed could bring trouble they stage a pre-emptive attack.

Patients with extremely serious conditions, or ones they perceive that way, occasionally ask for extrathorough answers, but no amount is enough. Unlike those who want to understand what they are up against, they fight off all understanding and keep everything going in frustrating circles. There's a component of, *Please wave your magic wand.* It is a very basic, childish reaction. It's like, if they make it enough of a bother for the doctor, then the doctor won't want to deal with it and will find it easier to just say, *don't worry, I can make it go away.*

There is no magic stuff that the doctor can open up for a few special people. When it is spelled out, this behavior is silly, yet it's all too easy to behave this way. It's nearly impossible to face up to it.

Some patients get angriest when it has to be explained to them that *there isn't a perfect, no compromise, no irritation, no effort, low (no) cost solution that will give them the ease and range of performance they once had.* Some bluntly say they will not leave until I give them a no-com-promise solution, and paying a penny extra for it would be a compro-mise: They make it clear that any compromise they pick will be returned with complaints.

The staff knows that no matter what they do now, they will get complaints. I tell them not to feel bad about it, and that they need not play along.[5] This person figures h/s'll pick one compromise then get the other choices free by complaining. If such a patient ever seems to have a legitimate problem, the best way to handle it is never to give anything new without taking back the first one—so they become the only people who can't collect an extra for free.[6] After an exchange they generally return crying the original compromise we had advised had been superior.

---

5.   If I do not own the office this is just a suggestion.
6.   The old "re-return and get them both free" trick.

As with *the boy who cried wolf,* when this patient has a real problem with any treatment or service it is hard to tell the difference.

A doctor's staff should be aware that some people return more often after being exposed. They do this to convince themselves that everyone has forgotten the obvious and now sees them as a good patient who deserves extra service. The con person has conned h/hself into submission. In the optical world they come in with complaints and request adjustments, and the experienced staff pacifies them by having them wait quite a while for the "major adjustment work" being done.[7]

The reality of any behavior is that it is a continuum, not a one or the other thing. Conpeople with hidden agendas are far to one side. People who want some information are in the middle. On the other end are people who don't want to hear anything.

One group in the middle are people who rattle off questions but won't listen to answers. They feel good about themselves for taking responsibility, but they miss the point: It's about the answer, dummy (Thank You President Clinton). They're the same type who feel good and healthy for buying a gym membership even though they'll never use it. As we've discussed, for going through the motions of an explanation so we all can feel we did our part, meaningless big-words and numbers can't be beat.

The world survives on meaningless numbers. There is truth in this joke I made in my first year out of school. *For doctors the most important thing they learn in school is the one thing they are told never to do there: how to "fudge"*[8] *numbers to get the right results.* Bureaucracies demand skill manipulating numbers.

There are some people who go out of their way to invite an explanation well aware that its basics would take years of schooling. They demand that the doctor explain why something is this way or a certain

---

7.   If you are now wondering whether you are being made to wait while little is really done, don't worry—unless you are also worried that you might have gone too far pushing for something—

8.   Curiously, another word for fudging results is "doctoring" results.

treatment is needed or why h/s must give up a food or activity. When the doctor can't explain simply and quickly they challenge on a basis that goes something like, *So there is no real reason I have to…*

Some people may ask for this depth because they want to be confused. They are torn between responsibility and being scared to know. In a movie they'd be told to pour a stiff drink and sit down. In reality they can ask for the complicated version. It's like looking it up in a foreign language.

◆   ◆   ◆

I want to turn the tables: How do patients answer questions during their case history? I know what you're saying: *This doesn't come up. My doctor doesn't really ask much and what h/s does ask is mindlessly recited from a list of standard questions. H/s doesn't really pay attention to the answers more than a tape recorder would.* Granted. In fact all the games some patients play are not the main reasons doctors don't take good case histories: They just don't. In school doctors are taught that it's extremely important—by someone who reads that information off in robotic fashion. You are officially assessed for quality of this skill early in your time as a clinician by a guy who robotically listens to whether you read the proper list of questions then properly recorded results for posterity, then moved on.

Furthermore, I have never in my life heard of anybody being held back for problems in their case history skills. Back in school I stunned more than one supervisor by "magically" knowing stuff about the patient nobody else ever knew. I asked! I dug. A good *Columbo* impersonation is better than $25,000 in sophisticated tests: It can provide answers before there's any other clue that these tests might even be needed.

Despite all of this, I will still turn the tables. We'll observe that rare bird, the *silver—stethoscope—billed, good—case—history—taking* doctor. When h/s does ask a question, the response may not relate to it at all. Even if generally applicable, it is often out of place and, at this moment, possibly misleading. People take insult when they give info in their order and the doctor wants it in h/h order. There are reasons for the doctor's order.

- Things make better sense in the proper order. If something comes up that needs further investigation, it can be checked later. The order can be frozen here if the doctor sees a need to investigate this point right now. That is not the same as moving off on a hundred tangents a patient happens to think of at the time that don't relate to the question.

- The proper order prevents things from being skipped! You wouldn't interrupt a flight mechanic on h/h pre-flight checklist. If you are getting to something you're sure will interest the doctor if h/s'd just give you the chance, get your ego out of the way. Cut the 20 minutes of BS and blurt what counts out at the top. If any more is needed it will come out in the questioning of the important part. Doctors have no time for this storytelling, so you'll never get to the point that would catch their interest. Even if you do, by that time they're just letting you ramble while they are doing real work. They may not catch the interesting part!

There are people who reply to any question by shouting *angry absolutes*. It might go like this: As an answer to a polite, "What do you see now?" a doctor might hear an enraged, "I don't see nuttin!" They are willing to sacrifice proper care for some agenda, even if all they want is more attention. It's amazing how people will put themselves at risk to be in control.

Most people who casually witness such goings on assume the patient is full of mistrust. Not quite. Mistrust causes manipulations to force the doctor to be more honest. These manipulations push the doctor away from the truth, and honest results become impossible. My guess is that their agendas are full time and have nothing to do with this moment. It is so worked into their behavior that they no longer pay attention to what it makes them do. Responding in this fashion only gets the doctor's guard up. H/s will be wary of doing anything. Because h/s can't trust this patient's own input, the doctor will never be confident enough to do much at all. This doctor is forced to leave things alone until the problem is big enough to make the patient cooperate, or until it is so distinct that it can be diagnosed with no assistance from the patient. Ironic, ain't it! If you speak in these "angry absolutes," a doctor may not help until there are absolute findings.

Another angry absolute is, *I don't wanna hear it.* This is usually from patients with very specific agendas. They will only accept the answers they have previously invented. Some include minor conspiracy theories. When they imply you are "BSing" them it is to protect their BS. These patients tend to be extremely dishonest, and they can't conceive of other people being much different: They truly mistrust anything you say since they are always untrustworthy.

Some have come up with their own diagnoses and treatment plan, and they view any alteration from this in conspiracy theory terms. Most are product oriented.[9] This might be because they are addicted to a prescription drug,[10] intend to give it to a friend who doesn't have coverage, or sell it. Anything that makes them jump to the conclusion that they won't get what they want causes fiery outbursts. It can also simply be a matter of someone who remembers[11] what they had and liked years ago and decides they want that. They even make their own adjustments to the prescription for small differences in their symptoms.

The angry, rude, and insulting, *I don't want to hear it,* would get this person kicked out, or worse, anywhere else. A doctor must soldier on. A common time to hear this is when a patient complains about "the

---

9.   These can combine due to paranoia and poor thinking so the patient's convinced h/s medically needs whatever h/s wants.

10.   Some will (aggressively) insist the doctor can get them illegal drugs.

11.   They are often remembering incorrectly to begin with. On the other hand, some people mention a recent version that is still viable as helpful information. We are not referring to these people.

system" while angling for things that are not available or applicable. If the doctor tries to correct h/h false understanding of the system so h/s can make better use of it, the bad patients quickly distinguish themselves from upset or worried patients by unleashing the aforementioned verbal assault.

There are people who push the doctor to help them with a lie, possibly to a criminal level. A simple example is the vision screening for renewing a driver's license. The performance most states require is very easy. On top of that, if somebody says "you failed," you probably failed by a significant margin. Incredible sympathy already biased the test in your favor because, frankly, nobody wants to get into this fight.

If someone finds out they have failed, the proper reaction should be concern for their eyes. Most people who fail already know they have a condition and have lost vision, so they aren't even curious.[12] They shout, *But then I can't drive.* That's the point: For everyone's safety they're not supposed to. The doctor already balanced guilt over other peoples' safety when h/s was lenient during the test; h/s will not be an accessory to vehicular manslaughter.

I've endured long harangues. The failure by these drivers is due to their limitation, but they act like it's my fault, so the least I can do to make up for failing them is to pass them. There have been threats, attempts to bribe me, and accusations of failing them in order to get a bribe. There have been promises that *I know I can't see, I really won't use the license.* That's an insult to my intelligence. If they're never ever going to use it, why are they going berserk for it? Some say they don't drive, but they attach feelings of independence to being able to drive. If you know you can't use it the license makes no difference. They want the license to maintain the option of driving, just in case. In truth there is intent to use it occasionally.

If such usages are as rare as these patients would claim, why not just drive illegally at that moment? That would be easier than getting a

---

12. Curiously, until such patients are told they can't drive, they love to complain about their terrible vision.

license illegally now! Their hidden reasoning is that if there's an accident, that crime is their fault. If they get me to pass them and then they drive and hurt somebody, the crime becomes my fault for passing them.

We retest them on our time, even letting them in free on other days trying every which way to see if they can do better. We point out that they are free to take the form elsewhere and try.[13] They never do. This may seem like an evil person: H/s is acting with annoyingly self-centered disregard for the lives of all others; however, this isn't an unusual person. It's a side that comes out to some degree in almost everyone. A small percentage of people have the inner strength to deal with such news completely rationally. Doctors accept this and put up with such behavior as part of the bigger "medical condition." Saintliness aside, improved communication skills really help here, even if it must be communication with relatives of the patient. It is amazing how many people with treatable conditions will go blind rather than go to a specialist, all while screaming that all would be well if we just signed the form.[14] Police get to see this side of normal people. Doctors see the same things, but don't have sidearms at the time.

---

13.   No form I've seen asks if you've ever failed, so you can go to many places. There's always some crook who will pass anybody. Few go elsewhere even if we offer to refund their exam fee to get rid of them. My guess is that when they do get into an accident they want it to be the first tester's fault. It's easier to shift feelings of guilt into blame that way. It's also harder to tell a judge the last person duped you into driving if the previous doctors testify to the truth.

14.   It is impossible to tell patients whose licenses aren't up for a couple years that they shouldn't drive. If you know you can't meet legal standards, you should stop driving now! Would you let someone who lost both eyes in an accident drive until license renewal time? As far as people in real life are concerned, if they got a license two years ago saying they were good for four years, then they're going to drive—over your dead body.

◆   ◆   ◆

For sheer frustration, nothing can match the patient who keeps changing answers. This is not changing an answer once in awhile or saying things that contradict each other; that's all of us at some point. These patients keep changing everything.

Every explanation gets a change in the complaint in order to keep the complaint alive. If their original statements were vague, any attempt to clarify things is taken as an attempt to alter their statements. They fight to change it back. Back to what? They just steer away from wherever they think things are heading. If this has you confused, imagine what it's like being the doctor living though this confusion.

Sometimes the original statements give an idea of a message. The first time the patient changes it the doctor figures the original statement just came out wrong. Assuming we do not believe the patient has lost h/h senses (a very real possibility in a medical setting), the second and third versions indicate the presence of a faker. The reasons any particular patient is doing this vary greatly, but the pattern is common. Spend one day as a doctor, you'll see it.

I only classify them as really frustrating when they meet two other conditions.

1. They get nasty and insulting about it, each and every time insisting they've never said anything but exactly what they are saying now.[15]

2. The doctor knows they have something serious, so h/s can't just say, *the heck with it,* and shepherd this patient out of the exam room.

---

15. They lose track and eventually return to saying what the doctor claims h/s heard them say, but they're still screaming that this is not what they had told the doctor.

Some patients have one story they want to push, but they alter the presentation to keep it going. They make the doctor go through all the time and work to test a complaint that just doesn't show itself in any way. It's impossible to prove something isn't there, and reasonable certainty may take a while. The doctor demonstrates all that has been found and not found, but this patient doesn't want to understand. Finally, upon realizing that they can no longer debate against the reality, these patients figure that it's time to beat logic by getting uncontrollably emotional. They want the doctor to take this as "proof" that h/s is magically wrong and go looking for their problem in "mystical" ways—or at least give them what they want out of having the imaginary ailment. Maybe they just think they can annoy the doctor into giving in. Some make sure they are heard all over the office to "soften" the doctor.

Many of these people behave this way all the time. They make one big mistake. They assume a doctor is the easiest victim for passive-aggression because h/s must sympathize and never appear to do otherwise. Actually, doctors live in a much more absolute world for scientific and legal reasons. Beside, as we've discussed, every patient is there for the doctor's sympathy, so h/s's immune to treating one special because they try for special treatment.[16]

Getting emotional never overrides medical reality: When it's used as a weapon it's a red flag. Doctors see serious causes of emotion all the time. They are especially attuned to real-life drama queens who use emotional collapses as weapons without even thinking about it. No doctor survives without a "blackbelt" in self-defense against passive-aggression.

---

16.   Doctors, however, are suckers for the patient who suffers bravely and makes a
      point of not trying for special treatment.

◆   ◆   ◆

Some patients have a little knowledge and use it to make any explanation an opening for a rough time. For instance, a patient might ask for a copy of their new glasses prescription then complain of something like *too much plus sphere*. They think they sound good enough to intimidate a doctor, but their limits of knowledge show through too quickly.

A related problem is patients who say, *tell me this,* to help them mold their exam responses. They're asking to help kid themselves. The doctor can't tell you anything that could impurify your responses. Some patients ask for general information about the test to figure out how to steer the proceedings. (Having that kind of information makes doctors terrible patients.)

◆   ◆   ◆

Some people just tell the doctor to examine them. This is like having a car with a rattle in the dash and just telling the mechanic to check out the car for problems: It's cheaper to buy a new car. It can be said as a challenge; some have actually shouted, *You're the doctor, you find the problem!* They feel it's the doctor's job to do everything, including figuring out the complaint. Some come in complaining about another doctor's prescription, but fail to bring the prescription along. That's like taking a bus to tell the mechanic about your car. Remember, you're not asking if you need medications, you're asking if you need a change. Without seeing what doesn't work you may be put right back on the same things. They may be the correct initial choice and your problem indicates a deeper reason that you must be treated differently: The idea that the first doctor was simply wrong is just one of many possibilities.

◆   ◆   ◆

Some patients feel that if they get the doctor into a long friendly conversation, they can ease h/h into giving them things. Questions are just one tool to start this. They're after product: Upgrades, items not covered by their plan, possibly even for a physician to violate clinic policy for them or to get drugs they shouldn't have. It's easy to separate them from people who happen to ask for something: When the answer is "No," are they still grateful for the thorough exam, treatment, and explanation, or does it ruin their total exam experience? People can be unaware of their own behavior this way. We don't necessarily plan to chat the doctor up to lead to favors: We are friendly to anybody when we are leading up to asking for a favor. If we succeed we see the favor as a small separate part, not the result of a manipulative strategy.

◆   ◆   ◆

To end this part of our discussion let's look at one peculiar bird. Some patients avoid giving any information because they fear being wrong. They can be another example of those who say "check me" but won't state the actual complaint. It is worse when they won't give answers that are part of the testing. They'll even stall to consider the answer when a doctor goes, "does this hurt?" and never manage to answer.

Testing for glasses is all about patient preferences. While every patient finds some choices difficult, these patients find every choice impossible. To get them at ease responding I'll give them something I estimate to be decent, and have them compare it with something so far off I might as well just cover the eye (I've even done that). Some say something seems wrong, but still won't pick the pretty good view over the covered eye! They are insistent that they are trying hard. To them, risking a mistake by ever giving an answer would be poor cooperation.

When these people are somewhat aware of their dynamic, they hit the doctor with a preemptive accusation that h/s should be more patient.

My own guess is that this is just an extreme version of a general problem. Many people want their health to be the doctor's job and doctors should leave them out of it: To take responsibility for one decision on the test is too much.

There's a bit of *Rodney Dangerfield* in the daily life of every person in any medical service. It's a vicious cycle, a problem in someone's head becomes reason, *to attack me, I tell ya, I don't get no…I should just learn to keep quiet, but I keep opening my mouth. I tell you, opening my mouth is like opening…*

Pandora's Box

5

Pandora's Box

Opening the lines of communication also opens this dangerous box. Some of the contents are from the special category of...

Vicious Cycles

Some are cycles of cause and effect, others are "Catch 22s" or self-defeating cycles of logic. For those who missed the movie; applying for a Section 8 insanity discharge from combat displays too much sanity to qualify. And now to your regularly scheduled programming...

◆   ◆   ◆

Patients spout many strange medical beliefs. Correcting these is difficult because the patient may have believed them for years. Some get angry because you have now insulted h/h self-image, parents, grandparents, favorite teacher, best friend, conspiracy theorist, or even cult leader. The doctor who can't resolve this is seen as untrustworthy and conniving.

Unless it is somehow immediately critical few doctors correct these assumptions. Letting h/h ramble on, however, is taken as confirmation of h/h views.[1]

---

1. Some will squeeze in their world, political, racial views, etc. If you don't fight them, they take it as "expert" support. If you disagree, you're suspicious or incompetent.

For example, many patients are certain an injury or medications caused their need for glasses. You only get grief for saying, *It's not from the injury, you just never checked before.* Millions of people have blur they think of as normal. I have checked with approximately 500 patients whose glasses allegedly came from an injury, but scientifically appeared unrelated, to see if they had a real eye exam within the 10 years before the incident: Almost all had not! The few exceptions were never positive, and even their possible exams would have been at least 5 years before the injury.

The only reason these patients never had glasses before was that they had avoided eye doctors. I present their cases for what they are; exams due to injuries in which *routine* needs for glasses are also uncovered. This is bad from their perspective for third-party coverage, lawsuits, workman's comp, disability, or even a good story. Many people who have avoided eye exams for years did so for self-image reasons. Injury glasses are a "battle scar," but they'll be damned if they'd take the insult of glasses for normal reasons.

It's okay to let them believe the glasses are from an injury if all that does is get them to wear the glasses. The truth, however, may not only be legally, but medically necessary. For example, this patient often has amblyopia: In supersimplistic terms, h/s went so long with one eye blurred that when glasses clear things up the brain has trouble dealing with it. A specialized training program might help. If I don't accept the patient's wrath in order to explain this, it goes on to be considered undiagnosed vision loss resulting from trauma. No amount of tests will find the nonexistent damage. I receive no benefit, and no compliment for a job well done, except in my own head. If the patient follows my advice and gets the vision back, they still figure they might have won the lawsuits and still somehow have regained their vision.

Most doctors understandably say nothing or resort to meaningless gobbledygook. Of course, if asked to be an expert witness doctors must spell out the reality. At that point the patient starts stories about how doctors are part of a conspiracy to prevent them from getting their due.

Our own taxes/premiums/investments ultimately pay for "their due." I am proud of straightening out such misconceptions, a stance that risked physical danger more than once. I use unique communication tricks to minimize the problems, so I'm still living and able to type.

◆   ◆   ◆

Doctors have their own bad theories, often of the chimp-and-hammer variety. They can't explain too deeply because it's a house of cards. When different medical fields overlap, these theories are used by each field to claim all potential patients are theirs.

We've discussed how doctors as a group aren't geniuses. They stand out in hard work and sacrifice for their studies. Insecure doctors may avoid "educating" patients to preserve their self-image of possessing some intrinsic specialness. It's demoralizing when a patient grasps things that took the doctor months of study. Despite any facade doctors can make no group claim to having super-secure personalities, in fact titles have an attraction for insecure people.

Possibly of more importance, patients are comforted by feeling that brain surgeons, like rocket scientists, are special. Rocket science isn't personal (yet), and even on a jet airliner you think about the pilot,[2] not any scientist. Brain surgery can become very personal. We feel safer thinking doctors are inherently different: Not subject to human failings. It's unsettling to realize that the people your life depends on are as fallible as you. It also protects some people's egos if they can see others as born for certain positions: There's no reason to regret why you

---

2.   Sign of the times: We think more about airport security than about scientists and engineers or even pilots when it comes to worrying about staying aloft.

didn't work to become something like this if they had to be born that way.[3]

Neither side loves the truth: Some regular people earned a certain status through harder work. Patients want to deify doctors for several reasons, and to some doctors this is music to their ears. These very patients may accuse doctors of playing god, but the cycle of deification often starts from the patient.

In more trusting times we worshiped doctors from afar. We still need to worship, but from up close where we can interrogate them. This is ostensibly to put one's mind at ease by proving the doctor is, well, godlike; however, when we investigate we'll only accept an answer of "not a deity" because our egos as equals are involved. It's a Catch 22: We want to induce the only answer we won't allow! The best solution is to silence the questions—like a god who need not answer.

◆   ◆   ◆

People ask why doctors don't just take a special course in creative talking for doctors. Simple. To develop it, doctors would have to get practice by talking more, but talking without already having the skill is risky. This cycle leads to a field with no researchers.

The same can be said of the "industry" from a top-down perspective: The system seems almost "set up" for limited communicators, and good ones have pressures to comply. This reinforces the system to select more limited communicators who thrive under the present conditions, which in turn makes conditions even worse for the good ones. We can't just start selecting for better communicators and throw them out there, the field they'll work in has to change to what it would have been had communication been supported all along. In that setup, a

---

3. Many people have prejudices favoring doctors of a race other than their own, and many women born before women were commonly doctors refused to accept women doctors. They are exhibiting this desire to see doctors as magical entities born to be doctors. The doctors, therefore, can't be like themselves.

bad communicator would have to improve to survive. As it is the payment industry would need a revolution to encourage and provide time for a quality communication. Patients would have to adapt as well. Hospitals and other institutions would have to overhaul their task-assignment and organizational structures.

Almost everybody believes most people are terrible drivers, but almost everybody counts themselves as the rare good one. Most doctors believe that most doctors have communication problems, but that they themselves talk fairly well. My impression is that very few don't care, but the vast majority have themselves convinced that they have already done something about it. They don't realize how many chances to improve things with better communication skills are missed everyday, and how many problems are started by poor communication technique. They just know they have all these problems and no time for communication mumbo jumbo. As we have discussed, everyone likes to pretend the ten second explanation, possibly containing intimidating or virtually meaningless big words and numbers, is a good explanation. Could this be the "good communication" many doctors believe they provide?

There are now some communication courses in schools or continuing education. I've heard the ones in school described as "useful to provide the instructor a job." Doctors have told me they make nice continuing ed. credits to sleep through. Part of this may be student disinterest; part may be that a standard communication course with a sprinkling of references added is not truly geared to doctors. Would you like to perform stand-up comedy with a communication course for training? Without working as doctors, communication experts have little clue what the tool of communication must do in the field. This cycles back to the start of this section, the need for researchers in the field, preferably supported by big institutions who would also be looking for ways to revamp their overall operations.

◆   ◆   ◆

Here's a paradox: Because doctors are officially in charge medically, institutions feel free to force them into bad practice. If something goes wrong because a file clerk switches something, the bosses who pressured, or simply hired, h/h take the fall. If they use "gun to the head" pressure on a doctor, however, they're in the clear because officially the doctor had the final say.

◆   ◆   ◆

What about the case where a patient complains and complains and is not diagnosed? We've seen that a cold is a cold until it doesn't run the right course, then it's the next most likely thing on down the line. Lung cancer turns up occasionally, but for those who wonder why that patient wasn't tested more right away, it's simple: If there is the slightest reason to test, they test; with no clue or subtle difference, they don't. Otherwise, we'd be tested for cancer and fifty other things every time we sneezed, just in case!

Aren't extra complaints a reason to test? It's not that simple. Say 1000 people have symptoms. Perhaps 200 will ignore it as long as possible, so let's assume 800 report at milder stages. Of these, 400 may be natural complainers, 400 would be more literal. Of each 400, assume 395 resolve easily; for 5 of each group it's more complicated. We are keeping things simple; in reality, there are many variations in the middle.[4]

Perhaps 30 of each group of 400 actually start with extra irritation. All 400 natural complainers act that way. Of each set of 5 truly bad

---

4.   Many people search themselves for any irregularities because they are going for an examination. They can no longer tell the difference between things they find because they are trying to find things and small but significant signs of the beginnings of trouble. Others refuse to show weakness by ever complaining.

cases to be, maybe 2 are also early sufferers: Future problems don't always provide previews. We have 430 people behaving like early sufferers, if we know which 30 are noncomplainers we can initiate extra tests on them at the start. So at best we get a lead on 2 of the 10 bad cases. Any complainer who slips into the extra test group will eventually cause grief over having been put through extra tests!

The rest of the complicated cases will return unresolved, accompanied by about 100 complainers whose problems have vanished, but who refuse to let that end things. With literal patients doctors know potentially annoying tests are necessary. In the hordes of returning complainers a few actual problems are buried. Some are found. Given thousands, a few will slip through. You hear about them, but never of the thousands who acted exactly the same but were spared millions of dollars of painful tests. You hear nothing of the other group being completely handled with a minimum number of patients having to endure extra tests. Once more with feeling, *don't cry wolf.*

So far, at least, the problems had a physical basis. Hypochondriacs might state a symptom then prevent anything that might reveal a lack of a "physical basis." They'll dodge questions, refuse certain tests, refute explanations, etc. Malingerers always do this. Some people with genuine problems are scared into negativity: They act exactly the same way. It is a Herculean task to separate the patient who sounds bogus from the actors. Testing everyone with such complaints would swamp the system. Just a few exaggerations can bog the system down, because infinite testing can't prove that what isn't there, isn't there. The fact is, some people will die because they blend with the hordes who just act that way; far more, however, would die if doctors didn't screen out bogus-sounding performances. As it is a few real cases are missed, the other way all real cases would get lost on line with the fakes.

Taken to the logical extreme, only fakes would survive the wait to get testing and "treatment," which is a scary thought considering this cycle; the easier it is to abuse a system the more abused it will be. If doctors accepted every complaint as scripture, then hypochondriacs, drama queens, the lonely or attention starved, and outright con artists would step up their efforts until 99% of all health care was devoted to them. We'd have a lot of bodies in the streets, but very healthy hospital populations.

Better communication skills would certainly help to find the extra problems concealed by noncomplainers. They would provide some help in spotting complainers and discovering when they coincidentally have a real problem. Someone with better communication skills should also be doing PR, people watching the news should understand things such as those mentioned in these past few paragraphs.

We only hear of tragic tales. We don't hear of the thousands of exaggerations, hallucinations, and fabrications a doctor uncovers in order to find and save all the others. The detective work to find some little nugget of information buried in the show of a drama queen never makes it into popular lore.

Being in the news doesn't make a story true. News agencies seek and even help create these stories. Weeks of coverage often suddenly stop with little or no mention that it was all a fake, or that the patient had misled the doctors, or had ignored doctor's orders.

It's a puzzlement! A Catch-22 within this cycle: There are bad doctors. Only a tiny percentage of them are caught even when other doctors alert the authorities. They don't worry about patients making accusations. Good patients treated badly rarely take significant action. Scheming patients seem to find good doctors to be easier marks than bad doctors. Lawsuits are difficult, and the worst doctors are prepared to battle. A good doctor would never get his good name back! H/s agrees to terrible settlements to avoid the process.

Here's a nasty side of the cycle: If a doctor does catch something early, it becomes something that never happened! Forget stories. Let's say you gave bad descriptions or avoided descriptions or gave drama instead of the real description, but the doctor coaxed out what h/s needed. You'd feel you were helpful and never know how amazing a job it was to save you from yourself. If you're informed that the doctor prevented a potentially fatal condition at an early stage you might take it as overcautionary, *I know, the worst case of everything is death.* Even if you accept this, it's not the "pulled from the flames" experience of being saved after you become painfully ill.

◆   ◆   ◆

Here's a cycle doctors cause. Many times symptoms are apparent but no cause is obvious. The faster the symptoms are alleviated, the less likely it is the cause will ever define itself.[5] Patients who push for immediate relief, or who make it difficult or unpleasant for the doctor to investigate more deeply, tend to ignite this cycle more often. Patients who are assumed to have many problems, such as those with other severe illnesses or the elderly, are also more likely to suffer.

There is no such thing as "you're just getting old" in the lists of medical diagnoses. There are many things that are common with advancing age. There are things that are just built up wear and tear that present technology cannot help. There is, however, always a specific cause. If after finding the cause a doctor advises that, "we can't do anything but soothe the symptoms," or "the procedure is far too involved to be worth the effort," that is legitimate. It is wrong to dismiss the search for any cause and just mask the symptoms because *it's an age thing.*

Medications used to mask symptoms cause other problems. They also interact with medications for other symptoms and the medications for the problems the first medications cause. The cycle is explosive, a couple of medications lead to being on dozens of medications for exotic syndromes and a patient who is barely alive. I have witnessed cases where a doctor who knew how to communicate with the patient (or their caretakers by this stage) and with all the previous doctors

---

5.   Patients also do this by over treating themselves before a doctor sees their problem. For instance, drown a red eye in "Visine," and it is hard to tell whether to treat for a virus, a bacteria, or an allergy, or if you were just tired.

stopped all of the medications and cured most of the problems. The lively patient was then examined and treated for a real problem or two, not just the symptoms.

◆   ◆   ◆

Patients ask for advice for things outside the doctor's field. If I say, *I'm no dentist, but my friend had a similar SOUNDING problem and it turned out that simply by doing yadda yadda, but see a dentist because you might have something different,* patients take it as more authoritative than had a beer buddy said it. Sure, I included, "see a dentist," but people figure, *doctors always tell you to see the doctor, it's just business, or nervous precaution.* If it turns out you should have seen the dentist as I advised it can become my fault that you did something else.

People don't take polite hints to drop the topic and doctors don't want to say, *Shut the heck up with things out of my area of practice.* Is it any wonder doctors seem not to be listening? They hear way too much between the lines.

◆   ◆   ◆

The last cycle of logic for now—We can intellectually decide that class divisions should be eliminated in one conversation. Millennia may not suffice to "reprogram" our nature. Someone will always be of lower status and will need the comfort of attributing this to a class system. The people who perceive themselves as the lower class, therefore, will always underline class divisions: The excuse of being born to one's lot covers all. This puts the joy in insulting anyone who tries harder to improve h/h lot in life: *Look who thinks h/s's the bloomin King/Queen. You're nothing but a.... (one of us).*

Even in America, with our "rags to riches" mythology, we actually need the comfort of feeling that *people who have it better are born to it, we do the work that keeps them there.* Any exception must have been crooked and abusive of people like us. It's better to honor celebrities as the best of the best because deep down we know we don't have to give them true respect. True respect doesn't come as easily as worship.

In a class system you can rebel against an upper class, people with real power who can make you sorry. We go one better: Because nobody is officially the upper class we find less formidable stand-ins for our little rebellions. Doctors, even out of the office setting, represent a safe symbol of authority to attack.

Some people are obsessed with "putting *The Man* in his place," and doctors are safe representatives of authority, even if "The Man" is a woman. When a doctor (or a teacher, manager, etc.) must take charge or state facts and instructions in lecture form, such a person distorts that into something offensive. For those on the edge looking to "take it out" on someone, this will set h/h off.[6]

A few doctors have told me they have described this dynamic in similar terms. Others agreed after we spoke. They may not use references to *class struggles*, but they confirm that they see the behaviors I ascribe to it.

All doctors know that they are sometimes treated badly because of the title, but they constantly hear how life must be perfect for a doctor. Resentment may lurk somewhere. They hear legends of the perks of MD license plates, but experience the reverse: People who scratch a car with MD plates act like the doctor should pretend nothing happened. To sum up the attitude, *You're rich and you're supposed to be selfless. You fix it.* A doctor is lucky when h/s isn't sued after being hit. No matter how clear it is that their client hit the other car, lawyers know they have a good chance to win a suit against a victim with a medical title.

---

6.   The most cowardly of these people show up *The Man, corporate division*, by abusing minimum wage stand-ins at the counter. Observe people who might be pleasant at a *Ma-and-Pa* store but who manage always to find trouble at a huge chain. Places with an ambiance that lets you imagine the presence of *The Man* really set this type off, so a *Starbucks* employee sees this more than one at *McDonalds.* I am not counting regular "testy" (overcaffeinated?) customers.

On TV you say "doctor" to get better seats when making reservations. Reality? It might get you bad service. I'm always incognito, so waiters attend to me several times while sharing their snide remarks about the doctor they've been ignoring. They'll shout across several tables, "I know, I'll get to you DOCTOR!" Try sending back uneatable food when the staff has decided you can afford to throw away money.

Doctors sacrifice the best decades of their lives for a "doctor-style" middle age. Even if they manage to get it, what do you think it sounds like to a doctor when people speak condescendingly of how lucky h/s is? The response may be subtle, but for some it's fueled by a Pandora's Box worth of reaction to abuse past, present, real, or imagined.

We know, therefore, that doctors don't simply have trouble communicating and explaining without using big words. There's also a lot of stuff going on in the doctor's head, and a lot of stuff going on in the patient's head. There are bad doctors, but as a patient you have bigger problems from bad patients who affect the regular and even great doctors. Then there are the systems we're all stuck with. By now you're asking, *So what's a patient to do?* It's about time you asked that question. The answers are already waiting in the next big chapter...

6

How to talk to Doctors

Pick the right doctor. This is much easier than fixing one you don't like. Have you ever heard of *Oprah* or *Dear Abbey* advising a woman to marry the bad choice she intends to mold? That's true of any relationship.

Avoid the strong silent type. Get the yacky one who can back it up. Ask yourself, *With whom am I trying to communicate?* Bad doctors aren't always less competent. They are always concerned with doing their "business" quickly then moving on. You'll never communicate with them, they are processing you too fast. Pick these guys/gals out.

As *Captain Kirk* would assure you: In life the game isn't chess, it's poker. It involves more than strategy. Beyond foreseeing possibilities you must be aware of the odds of each. It involves bluffing and reading people. Mastering the subtleties can occupy lifetimes, yet this simple guideline will instantly prepare anyone to play:

Every game involves several players planning to make money off of another player. You must pick out that player. It's easy. Look around. If you can't pick h/h out instantly, then it's you. Leave. Run. Flee.

And always remember, a pro is the master on h/h turf. H/s lets you think you've done well when it suits h/h.

Make an effort to pick a competent doctor who inspires your trust and with whom you "relate" well. Switch when you must. All the following suggestions are designed to help good patients talk to good doctors. Don't waste your time trying to train a terrible communicator.

So…You've Entered A Doctor's Office

As mentioned earlier, the doctor is on the job for long hours working very hard with extraordinary demands upon h/h. This situation, however, is still repetitive to the extreme. H/s is bored. If you had to interrupt a busy office clerk you'd be aware that h/s wants to get h/h work done as fast as possible, protect h/h break time, avoid new problems and survive the boredom. H/s may feel unappreciated. Interruptions are problems until proven otherwise. You relate to h/h state of mind easily.

Approach a doctor relating to h/h state on this same level. To put the office clerk at ease you'd approach in a manner suggesting you respect h/h time. You'd make it clear that you are not going to add to h/h problems or burdens, and that you appreciate h/h help. You'd try to compliment h/h or make h/h feel good in some way. If you could make h/h laugh, all the better.

Once upon a time I experienced a strange sensation in my arm. I figured there was nothing to do for it, but it came up in a conversation somehow and I agreed to have it checked.[1] I had to visit several doctors, several times, for them to be satisfied that it was no big deal. As I met each one I managed to make some joke about the nature of my alleged injury and how I might have managed to cause the condition. I included something to the effect of, *so now my silly thing is interrupting your busy day.*

When each doctor would start telling me about a test that might hurt I joked about it in a way that <u>clearly</u> said, *it's okay and I accept that the discomfort is mine to deal with.* Few patients let the doctor know they understand that the painful test is what they need. Some patients give off "vibes" of disappointment or resentment. A surprising number of patients blatantly try to make the doctor feel guilty about making them suffer through tests.

---

1.   Doctors even have mothers like other people…the kind who make them go to
       doctors.

With one doctor, who seemed a bit off, I said, "You concentrate on the test and the results and I'll handle the pain part." He instantly seemed smooth, the test didn't hurt much, and I became a favorite patient. This one sentence demonstrated logic, responsibility, guts, respect for him as a person and as a professional, and knowledge that my welfare is in my hands rather than on his shoulders. Nothing advances your relationship with a doctor quite as well as assuring h/h that any unavoidable discomfort is yours with which to deal.

Because doctors actually come from Earth, they can have families. They get to spend much less time with theirs than you probably can with yours. Some are workaholics, which may have led them to become doctors in the first place; others are just swamped. The idea that a doctor might be more concerned with h/h child's coma than your child's scratch is alien to some people. Many pay lip service claiming to understanding that their doctor has human problems, but this has no effect on their actual behavior. Make sure you treat the doctor with the understanding you'd naturally have for any other person.

If a doctor seems particularly rushed, do what you would do to work well with any other human. Don't deny h/h right to feel rushed. Be patient, show h/h you want to help smooth things, and that you are not going to make a federal case that you think h/h rush is affecting you. H/s isn't skimping. If h/s could skimp h/s wouldn't be so rushed. I have found that if I try to hide the rush people look to make trouble, but if I make it clear that there are rushed circumstances (and I am making a heroic effort) very few do anything but express gratitude.

Here's one more *Catch-22*. You are trying to be unnoticeable on a day when everyone stands out as a problem case—and you want to be noticed for this. How do you get noticed for not being noticed? It's an art. There is no simple instruction, but maybe with practice…

◆   ◆   ◆

Don't try to be an entertainer if you are not entertaining. Be amusing or intriguing or interesting to a level you are actually comfortable with. When talking be open and brief. A doctor takes risks being friendly; prove you are not the one to worry about. Be careful—many people who have thought of this on their own do all the wrong things.

- Don't try too hard to prove anything.

- Never even seem to take control, not even control of getting communication itself going.

- Make it clear you are comfortable letting h/h be in charge.

- Let h/h feel that you won't abuse any information.

- Show that you won't panic and that you have the intelligence and determination to comprehend, but that you'd never use it to interfere.

- It must always be obvious that you would never abuse the privilege of time.

To prove these things, first and foremost don't do anything to indicate otherwise, including making any grand attempt to prove any of these things.

How can you demonstrate your intelligence without showing off some expertise? In your questions, your answers, and interested demeanor; never by shoving it in h/h face with big statements and non sequiturs.

People confuse demonstrating intelligence with showing someone up. That's about fair because as a society we confuse rudeness and insults for comedy and wit, and loud arguments for clever writing. It's actually easier to demonstrate intelligence without showing any knowledge at all. People view anyone who waits for their opinion as being wise.

Deferring to a doctor's position puts a doctor at ease. How you handle the information the doctor gives you is a key to getting more of it. Show eagerness and focus. Saying thanks for clearing something up is more than polite—it shows comprehension. This doctor enjoys being your guide now, so h/s tells you more. If you knew something, don't mention that in lieu of saying thanks. Avoid showing the doctor up by pointing out the next level. Turn such knowledge to your advantage by using it to "grasp things" h/s teaches you. Trying to impress the doctor by displaying "knowledge"

- makes it a competition.

- raises a warning flag that you might have an agenda

- makes h/h worry that you might be too opinionated

If you want to demonstrate such knowledge to intimidate a doctor you don't trust, don't be a fool, find one you do.

There is an exception when dealing with an uncommon, long-term, major problem. This often comes up with parents of children with unusual syndromes. Concerned parents often become obsessed with the field and know many more specifics than a doctor might. How does one handle this?

This can separate great doctors from good and not-so-good ones, and it has nothing to do with having encyclopedic knowledge of every possible condition.[2] It's about not being threatened by this. Unfortunately, conceding a lack of infinite knowledge makes a doctor vulnerable.

This can be easier if you have a long-term relationship with a doctor. Speak of research you have been doing since the doctor put you on

---

2. That's what encyclopedias and web search engines are for, but I wouldn't want to be treated by either one.

the right path. If you are seeing a doctor for the first time but you already have researched this condition,[3] don't show it all off at once. Follow the same old guideline: You can show a little knowledge, but it's always wise to ask for any good reference sources the doctor can advise. Don't say, *been there researched that;* just write them down and say thanks. If there are things you feel h/s should be told, do it diplomatically. Don't lecture—tell them you need their take on some information. It is even better if you can hand them a paragraph or two to read: If only from an acting standpoint, it is easier for you to maintain the proper receptive attitude when you don't feel you are teaching.

This isn't simply about manipulating h/h ego; it's about research help you need. I have seen very intelligent people do years of research that resulted in misconceptions due to some lack of basic knowledge of how to do research, or how to understand and incorporate it. There's often some nonsense a person reads and accepts early that wastes years of work afterward.

A lot of what you read is not entirely correct, to say the least. Get help figuring this out. The first choice should be your doctor. If h/s can't help, then it may be time for h/h to refer you to the proper expert. If h/s simply dismisses your properly diplomatic attempts to get legitimate assistance, then *mission control, we have a problem.* It might be time to trade h/h in on a new doctor.

Always treat the doctor like the expert, it puts h/h at ease. The problem with never having a magic moment of becoming a doctor is that self-doubt can always pop up. Keep them convinced that they can work wonders. Coach the doctor into wanting to crash through walls

---

3.   This can imply that you self-diagnosed it or that you switched doctors. A know-it-all who switched doctors is to be avoided. Your switch may be due to new coverage or a new home, but showing off what you know is still a bad choice for first impressions. Let them think they are doing a better job of getting you to the right information sources than anyone else did. Don't put down a previous doctor; just be very appreciative of this doctor's efforts. Seeing a specialist doesn't count as a switch, nor should the specialist have a problem with your level of knowledge.

on your behalf. If you can't because you have no faith in h/h ability, then once again, maybe you've chosen the wrong doctor.

No doctor knows more than a "millifraction" of the quadrillions of bytes of medical information. It is sometimes a Herculean achievement just to figure the right specialist to consult. A doctor has not the time nor the obsessive motivation to get into each and every thing.

Obnoxious people and fools "advise" doctors all the time. Great doctors overcome the resultant defensiveness to provide a chance to distinguish your input from theirs. They can use such input to help choose tests and find the treatment course, or to steer you to a specialist.

It is your duty to assist the doctor, but do this without showing h/h up for lacking infinite knowledge. Never make a statement sound like a challenge, and if possible gift-wrap the statement in a question:

> *NEVER: I studied the literature on this from the obscure disease of the month club and according to them you are completely wrong.*
>
> *AVOID: I've read up on this. Let me explain to you what's actually going on.*
>
> *BETTER: I've studied literature on this and according to the most respected, most often quoted sources they say...*
>
> *BINGO: I've been very concerned so I've been doing a lot of reading on this, I even brought one or two pamphlets. Do you think this could have something to do with me? What do you think of this (or could you explain this, it has me worried.) Do you think this is worth looking into? Can you advise me as to who I would need to see if it's this?*

The last choice labels you as an intelligent, cooperative, and concerned-but-not-panicky patient. Your doctor realizes that you are making the job of taking care of your health easier for h/h, and h/s both loses all defensiveness and is probably motivated to go the extra mile. H/s may want to make your call for you and learn more about this specialty h/hself.

◆   ◆   ◆

We've covered how graveyards are full of people who said, *It's my body, I know best.* The proper version is, *It's my body so the ultimate choice and responsibility is mine.* You come for expert advice because you don't know; if you want to turn it down or get a second opinion, fine. When doctors tell you things of a factual nature, debating the science just makes you look foolish. If you want to challenge a statement of medical fact about a known condition or specifics of each treatment, become a medical researcher.[4] A diagnosis can be questioned by another doctor and treatment plans certainly vary—even one doctor may offer several choices. You can also go to a quack or charlatan. You should be wary of friends who push you in that direction.[5]

---

4.   Calling medical science "wrong" is very different from asking about it's limitations. By simply looking back a decade we can see how many things treated to the best capabilities of medical science can be diagnosed and treated in geometrically superior fashion today. Brilliant researchers may become obsessed with improving the knowledge base for conditions they've experienced; however, in the moment these researchers would be the last to suggest just throwing out current medical opinion. They use the best known treatment to help them get back to the lab to work on bettering the treatment. Legends of them treating themselves refer to their need to test a possibility, not their confidence in the superiority of the untested treatment.

5.   Make sure the person advising you to go for "non-western" medicine isn't in your will! The world is teeming with people who have ancient, natural, and superstitious cures. They beg for Western medicine and have a life expectancy measured in dog years without it. Cures, like penicillin, have been stumbled upon over the millennia and many are buried in the lore and superstitions of the world's cultures. Scientifically based ("Western") medicine has always learned from these sources and is doing so more actively than before. However, for every folk remedy with a basis in fact there are hundreds that are useless or harmful. Even those that work are rarely very effective. Scientific method figures out how and why things have an effect, isolates, emphasizes, and assists the active ingredients and produces treatments with hundreds or thousands of times the efficacy yet with fewer, milder side effects.

A second (third, fourth?) opinion might not be covered. To avoid paying, some patients fake accusations against the doctor so the next guy is considered to be the first, covered, opinion. If insurance is involved, you can get on a very real list for this fraud.

Some patients fight the doctor to the literal death to deny things exist; for instance: *I don't have diabetes, you just want to charge for a lot of tests and then for treatment. I DON'T HAVE IT!* Need I tell you not to fight a doctor who says you have something?

This does not mean you can't ask for a retest or a second opinion. On the other hand, relax when you are told, "relax, it's nothing." This is always right. Almost. Relax anyway. Don't look for symptoms because then you'll always find some, real or not. If a real one shows up, you don't have to be on the lookout, it will announce itself. Then go tell the doctor.

◆　　◆　　◆

And now the mysterious secret to not crying wolf:

You must not even seem like a wolf crier. If you have complaints that can't be pinned down, be aware of how things look to everyone else. Many bad choices can be avoided just by staying aware of this. I can see a hypochondriac many times without labeling h/h a wolf caller, but I've spotted others as wolf callers the minute I met them. Definitely go to the doctor with every tiny concern. Report them logically. Don't play for sympathy to cover lack of visible evidence. Bring even the tiniest problem, but don't dramatize even the biggest. Adding extra symptoms backfires because when they are dismissed some real ones might go with them. The more dramatizing involved, the fuzzier the line between fact and act.

Never calculate the right amount to say. Simply describe anything you've felt or noticed. Don't look for sympathy or to place blame or to get things off your chest: *Just the facts ma'am.* Don't leave anything out that you think might mean something, but don't kid yourself that whining, complaining, and exaggerating are facts.

Doctors are very attuned to when they are getting just the facts and when they're not. They can weed out certain things that don't matter. When you stray too far they can't separate the facts, lies, and hyperbole. They eventually dismiss you as a source of help on your own behalf.

Stories are more fun to tell than to hear. Being pressed for time and feeling trapped makes listening even less pleasant. If you ramble, the doctor is thinking, *shut up already.*[6] A couple story breaks cause your doctor to avoid giving you another opening. Save your talk for something important to say. If you're truly that amusing, the doctor will get you to talk.

If we waved a magic wand and made things perfect, you'd still feel something wrong if you thought about it. We can never test to perfect certainty anyway. A doctor can only investigate what calls out to h/h. Remember, the more a voice calls, the less it calls out! When the boy called wolf, at least only a limited area had to be checked for one thing—a large ferocious canine. As a patient you may be asking for infinite things to be looked for in infinite ways. If the need to bend the doctor's ear isn't absolutely medical rather than a need for attention, to complain, or hypochondria, you will eventually be the one to suffer your consequences.

If nothing wrong can be found, but you are sure that something is going on beyond the doctor's senses, be logical about the possibility of more tests. Do not plead emotionally, "But there's really something wrong!" If you are right you'd feel exactly the same as millions of mistaken individuals. Doctors "hear" the calm, logical request much more clearly. If they still can't find anything, return if more symptoms

---

6.   I have told patients to shut up already, you're interfering...but I was incredibly charming. I really do talk to patients in the open and free way I describe in this book, except without benefit of editing and no pause for a breath. If I was your normal medical person this book wouldn't exist.

appear: If it's real and becoming serious it will eventually become detectable. Unfortunately, there are limits to what we can diagnose in time.

Unless you are reading this after the fall of civilization, present technology can find things in minutes that took weeks just decades ago, at earlier, more treatable stages. On the other hand, compared with thirty years from now we are probably hopelessly crude.[7] When nothing shows up it means nothing SHOWS UP. You should relax, but don't fall asleep at the wheel. The only part you can control is being able to return to be monitored without any "wolf crier" label to bog things down. Many people live long lives and have made that emotional plea a thousand times. The rest of us never do, or maybe once. Save it for the day you'll need to be believed, or the cost could be your life.

"The fault lies not in our stars but in ourselves"[8]

Do not preach from a lofty position. Anything beginning, *This is important,* when *hello* or *do you want me to sit here* is appropriate, should be avoided. Never greet a doctor with accusations of what another doctor did. Entering a new office on the attack doesn't make you seem to have been victimized in the past. Even if you can convince the doctor of it, it makes a terrible, lasting impression. It seems plausible that you mistreated those doctors leading to the problems in handling your case.

Accusations about other doctors ending with *but you're good* are not a compliment. In caveman terms, when patient says, *you good, others bad,* doctor hears, *I leave, I say you bad also.* To a new doctor it indicates that the complaining is so out of control you can't even wait to

---

7. In *Star Trek IV* the crew comes back to our time and in a hospital *Dr. McCoy* comments on our most advanced techniques, "My God, it's the Spanish Inquisition." It would be nice to have his diagnostic tools. Less than two decades later some of the things that offended him already look primitive!

8. William Shakespeare said something like this.

get a feel for how this doctor will take it. This is not to be confused with a patient who has experienced at least part of an exam and says h/s prefers the new doctor without any specific complaints about any others.

A patient who comes in attacking the medical system is like a blind date who starts off by saying that all guys are bad.[9] Logic dictates that the one constant in all of those bad dates was her. There are three possibilities.

1. She's an angel with a real jinx. Even accepting this near impossibility, why should I suffer her present attitude?

2. She seeks out bad types. Well, then, coming here was an accident. It won't matter; she'll lose interest and go to what she seeks. In the meantime, why suffer her insanities?

3. She is the source of the trouble. Bingo. It is irrelevant whether she just blames her victims or causes them to react badly. Whether she was hurt once long ago, resulting in her becoming an ogre, is history. Discretion is the greater part of valor, coat please…

This patient is no different; the advice is the same. Change yourself, then find a good doctor and spare h/h your past. If a date told you that every date h/s ever had was miserable, you wouldn't think, *Here's my chance to be a hero and show her/him what a date with a great person is like,* you would think, *This is trouble, how fast can I escape.* So, guess what a doctor is thinking…

◆   ◆   ◆

If you believe you can be squeezed in, work to streamline your own exam; otherwise, in the exam room you will feel less rushed, and you

---

9.   Sorry ladies but I can't speak of the experience of dating a bitter guy.

will slow things. If you realize you do need full time, ask to reschedule; otherwise, this one exam may cost your favored patient status.

◆   ◆   ◆

Avoid saying, *if there's no charge I would like…* as if you were considering a refill of your soda. We know that's what people mean. At least leave room to imagine a sense of propriety is operating. Ask, *Do I need it?* If you do, the charge shouldn't matter; if you don't, then it's abuse of the office or the coverage. If the doctor says you need something "sooner or later," it's fine to decide *not now* after hearing the price. If, while you're deciding, you're told it's covered, it is fine if you say, *Well then I don't have to think about it; let's do it.* Forget the notion that all doctors make fortunes[10] pushing every possible covered item. Most doctors are not fans of people who abuse coverage.

Wanting things only if they are covered indicates the attitude of, *I am the responsibility of the doctor and the insurer and the government, but not my own responsibility.* You're holding your health hostage for handouts, like it should matter to everyone but you.

◆   ◆   ◆

Your first words should never be "you were wrong." Even if h/s was wrong, you might as well say, "pistols at ten paces." Everyone gets defensive when accused, but doctors have much more to fear from admitting any imperfection to a troublemaker.

People who enter on the offensive tend to be those who do it for attention or the joy of complaining, so the complaint itself actually carries less weight. Before bringing up a real problem settle in, then be polite. Don't back the doctor into a position where agreeing that you

---

10.   A crooked doctor wouldn't leave profits to chance—you'd get no option. This also prevents "complications" because you won't realize these were anything but absolutely mandatory.

need assistance can be used against h/h later. State the symptoms objectively, let the doctor put any labels on it.

Doctors will make little mistakes just like you do and will correct them, but many have been crucified for innocent human failings that caused no great harm. There have also been cases where all harm could have been prevented had a "victim" honestly wanted help instead of lawsuit fodder. The doctor can often legitimately defend what was done: That's the nature of art. Don't force h/h to "focus" on the benefits of the treatment with which you are having trouble.

Just as there are complainers, there are people who truly "can't complain." Some people make it clear they will not tolerate complaints, whereas others invite abuse. Smoothness of interaction depends more on the mix of these qualities than the reality of problems. The old fashioned "I am God" doctor rarely drew complaints. Their descendants are accused of behaving as they actually may have, whereas we look back at their days as a golden age when every doctor was a "Marcus Welby." The friendly house-visiting doctor disappeared exactly the same time as the last of the *Godlike* doctors faded from the scene. Could it have been that our fear of one type gave the other type the freedom to be so open?

Complainers manage to annoy everyone everywhere, but they are drawn to doctors (and clergy) who tend to listen politely when they know someone is a whiner spouting stories. Some apparent hypochondria is actually a fondness for complaining or a conscious play for attention.

You must check yourself with any complaint: Is complaining the goal or do you want to have a good doctor who will help your real problems? Then play poker: Stop complaining about every doctor so you can learn to tell the bad ones from the good ones. Until you do, the habitual complaining will make the good doctors you cannot spot act like the cold, distant doctors.

If you are clear on your goals, you likely have a gameplan. Get them out of your head and get into the doctor's head. Delete notions that doctors must act in doctor ways: What would be in your thoughts if you had to hold in your reactions behind a professional facade? People try things all day long and you'd be simmering, then someone thinks they'll fool you with something you've seen thousands of times. Can't they at least be less boring! Now, how should someone break through your shields and nudge you without setting anything off? I'd try to appease you even if you appeared calm, because that calmness could be the eye of the storm.

Some doctors neutralize the pressures by dehumanizing patients: subintelligent beings who can't be held accountable for annoyances, literally beneath contempt. This may be behind your feeling like "a piece of meat." I know of a few doctors who treat people like meat because they are terrible doctors. I can't count all the doctors who to some degree have discounted people to keep from "going postal."[11] No direct assault can get such a doctor's real attention. Consider how to ease into the real attention of a mind in this mode.

◆   ◆   ◆

Doctors do something so important it is power. We feel weak in turn, so we do things to undermine that power. This is very bad timing, seeing as this is right when we need the help of such power. Preventing this takes constant self-vigilance; minuscule resentments can sabotage the relationship.

◆   ◆   ◆

Never claim knowledge of what the doctor's "trying to pull" because it's like some other doctor you caught. Don't even entertain such notions in your head: It will show through. It can also lead to figuring, *I've decided the last guy BS'd me, so if this guy doesn't tell me what I want*

---

11.   Apologies to postal workers, but that word unfortunately now best conveys the intended meaning.

to hear I'll challenge it and h/s'll back down 'cause I will have bluntly called h/h out.

If two doctors do the same thing, either they found a genuine problem, or you've somehow stumbled onto two in a row who pull the same exact thing the exact same way. You probably have the condition, so your resistance is risky. Poker 201: It isn't a question of whether one-in-a-billion things happen; they happen once in a billion times. Never risk anything on them.

If you're certain that your case is the one in a billion, challenging a crook within h/h field of expertise can be hazardous to your health, and identifying the other doctor gives them a chance to coordinate their stories. Just do a better job checking out a third doctor and let the authorities check out the first two.

Don't make a doctor suffer for your previous relationships. Trying to force the helpful one into doing even more to make up for your past can only backfire. This doctor will do the minimum acceptable amount to process you out. Because actions talk loudest, this doctor now figures that you abused the previous doctor and staff and caused your own problems. If you truly were mishandled that's between you and that doctor or your lawyers. Never bring it up to the next doctor. Whatever you must mention as part of the medical history should be stated factually. If unavoidable, say the past doctor made this mistake or that mistake; check emotional baggage and accusations at the door. Avoid anger, and no playing the sympathy card. A doctor can tell when you've been mishandled and will go above the call of duty to help if you suffer in silence. Whining about past treatment invariably leads to scaring this doctor into h/h shell.

People assume that all a doctor has to do is work harder to "go above and beyond" on their behalf. More than likely it involves stretching the rules or even violating guidelines and policies of the institutions, insurance companies, etc. Doctors can't risk going out of their way for an aggressive person, even if the behavior doesn't directly bother the doctor: When they become this person's target, everything must be on record, by the book.

◆   ◆   ◆

People who squeeze onto a loaded schedule will then wonder why the wait is so long. Squeezing even includes saying "now" when told "you can get an appointment next Wednesday or squeeze in now." If there was room they wouldn't say, "squeeze in," or mention Wednesday. They probably already felt pressured to include the offer, but they're warning you by mentioning a real appointment.

You have a right to complain when:

1.   Your appointment was made in advance, and

2.   You signed in well before the appointment time, in time to have all paperwork done before your slot. Being nearly at the bus stop before your time slot ends is not on time. Bus broke down? How fascinating that it happens to the same people every time—maybe they bring gremlins along? [12]

3.   Special Note: Don't assume you have a right to whine when after a long wait you are told that the doctor left on an emergency call. If it is the first time, well, it's a doctor, emergencies happen. Be understanding and the staff might try to make it up to you somehow. If emergencies happen many times, then either the staff is "covering" or this is a doctor whose real work is the emergencies. Some doctors shouldn't schedule regular appointments! With

---

12.   Yes, once in a very rare while it happens to people who work to be prompt, the ones who leave a safety margin for traffic and flat tires. It's a funny thing, they come in apologetic and make it clear they know they are not entitled to their appointment. They ask if they should reschedule or if by luck there is an opening. They are grateful if they can be seen.

either reason, avoid this doctor. Don't waste your breath complaining about them in their own waiting rooms.

◆   ◆   ◆

Never tell a doctor you should get a certain prescription. You can ask if h/s thinks you have something and what h/s thinks about a certain medication. The moment you demand the doctor authorize what "Dr Yourself or Your Friend" has prescribed, all the doctor wants to do is get out quickly while doing as little as possible. Your complaints have naturally lost believability.

So, You Want to Build a Personal Relationship with your Doctor

Then it's time to inspect your goals. A doctor might become personal friends with a patient. H/s is generally not looking to do so. Some doctors will not deal with a person as a patient anymore if they've become too close.

As a rule you don't gain what you need by trying to be treated as a pal. In fact, because it's impossible to treat every patient better than the rest,[13] h/s is on the lookout for people attempting to rise above the others in some way. It is okay if a doctor senses that you are trying to mold a relationship if the message h/s sees is, *I'm trying to show you I'm a pleasant, cooperative, intelligent, and maybe even interesting patient.* H/s should not sense, *I'm trying to convince you that I'm a buddy who you'll treat better than your other patients.*

If you were to succeed you wouldn't think that you got more than you deserved; therefore, the implication is that others got less than they deserved. I've lost money giving glasses to certain patients who

---

13.   The doctor definitely can't afford to be perceived as treating any one patient better than the rest.

couldn't afford what they needed because in the particular case I decided to do so. I may have felt that each of these patients proved h/s deserved a break. It still was "a break"—they were not entitled to have me sponsor them. Doctors do these things all the time, but never for people who show that they assume they are entitled to it.

Some people just go in and strike up the perfect relationship as if it had always been there. It's natural for them. Even being fake is natural for them and comes off naturally. They aren't reading this book. You can't fake it. So, to start, stop being artificial with doctors.

It is not a good time to concentrate on striking up a better relationship when discussing your condition. If h/s pulls you into a consulting room afterward and indicates h/s has time to chit chat, then go for it; otherwise, you are forcing it and forcing h/h to guard the time. You'll take this as rudeness. Congratulations, you have succeeded in preventing a good relationship.

Just state questions and answers briefly and listen politely. Let h/h feel awkward with the silence, that will pressure h/h to talk. Absolutely never force talk while h/s's concentrating. Censor any feeling that you can decide to talk because you are the center of the attention, realize the "project" you will bungle for h/h is your health. People talk at the weirdest time: "Be *wery, wery* quiet!" The doctor has to concentrate and remember many details until they're recorded. H/s may be listening to something. Talking may also cause physical movement of whatever's being examined.

Using a doctor's first name shows disrespect for the doctor and the situation. It's also a key ploy of conpersons: When a salesperson starts calling you Joey or Suzy instead of Mr./Ms. you know to watch out for a tactic. So does a doctor. If h/s's a friend still don't use the first name until specifically told to. If nothing else you want them in the mind of seeing you as a patient rather than fooling around with a buddy. If you bump into your doctor socially, h/s is still "Doctor" until h/s tells you otherwise. You have the right to be peers outside without asking permission, but if h/s hasn't deemed that h/s can switch back and forth with you, then you may gain a friend but lose a doctor.

Power Plays

Never sit in on an exam without asking the doctor, that is a form of assuming control. No matter how justified the request, make the request, just like you would ask permission to do anything at someone else's house. The answer might obviously be, *of course,* but if someone forgot to ask you would wonder about the personality that feels so entitled h/s could forget to ask. Some forget, many feel asking is beneath them: They feel equally entitled to interrupt, another form of control. Interpreters, for example, and parents of younger children should come in, politely. Ask where to sit/stand instead of taking charge of the domain. Parents should not "help" the doctor unless specifically asked to do so.[14]

Unless you yourself are an emergency worker, shut your beeper off. Do not even leave the cell on so you can say, "I'm in the doctor's office, call later!" Shutting it off is message enough. People get into actual conversations; they expect the doctor to bust a gut for their benefit while they have more important things to do.[15] They steal a free extension out of the doctor's and other patients' time. If they explain how sorry they are that someone called them and the doctor says "okay," it's more like "okay, I'm ready to move on and get you the heck out of my way." They've just added insulting the doctor's intelligence to the list.

---

14. Many children do well until parents start giving them answers, correcting imagined mistakes, making them nervous, or even punishing them. Any attempt to protect the integrity of the exam results in the parent's wrath being unleashed upon the doctor. Such parents don't yell because there's bad behavior and don't correct because there was a mistake: They yell because they are angry and immature. They make corrections to appear to know something or to be in charge. They don't fool the doctor and they rarely fool the children.

15. There's always someone foolish enough to defend the fools. I won't waste time debating silly alternative explanations. What counts is that to the person examining you it comes off as offensively self-serving.

It isn't the caller's fault for calling; it's the fault of the person leaving it on.

◆   ◆   ◆

After asking a question you may fine tune it or ask for elaboration. You can ask the exact same question a second time. A third time might make you seem dense. It probably shows that you're not listening. It may seem that you'll keep asking until you get the answer you want.[16]

When a doctor's advice ends with your turn to make a decision don't badger the doctor to make your decision for you. H/s has already given h/h advice by this point, and nobody can make your decision for you. It's sometimes a lifestyle decision. The doctor's expertise covers how to do whatever you choose to do.

One type of decision that stands out is surgery. I prefer doctors who see it as a distasteful, last resort; I invented the saying, *Violence is the last resort of the incompetent and surgery is as violent as it gets.* When it is the only hope, well, logically there is no need for a decision, your dilemma is only emotional. When it is described as the clearly superior, but not the only choice, then you have to weigh all of the facts and the emotional part is one of the factors. Surgery is often optional, or elective. If you even think this is the case and you ask your surgeon if h/s would do it in your case, also ask how many surgeries of any type h/s ever had. Then ask how many bad injuries or conditions h/s has had where someone might have used surgery? Guess what. Surgeons avoid having surgery as much as possible.

Some patients who avoid decisions are our old friends who want to try one thing, then change their minds and claim it's the doctor's fault and collect all the choices for free. A doctor is much more likely to go

---

16.   With anyone, if a question hasn't been addressed after a second asking, it's foolish to ask the same way a third time. The second time shows you know it wasn't answered. Unless you know your question is inappropriate, being direct is fine, for instance, *You appear to be avoiding this question, is there a reason?*

above the call to help someone who makes the decision and returns taking full responsibility for their change of heart.

One more thing about lifestyle considerations: Specialists tend to be terrible with them. They look at surgery versus medication and other life-or-death-level things. The daily discomforts of living with the condition are not in their priorities. It's sometimes easiest just to return to your own physician with those questions. People want the answer from the specialist partly because they see them as superior doctors overall. Actually, to specialize is to simplify! They eliminate as much scope of practice as possible, and that may include communication skills. Perhaps there should be a communication superspecialist coordinating all other doctors.

◆   ◆   ◆

When caught lying don't pretend otherwise and don't make big excuses. People lie to doctors so often that it's expected. You've lost some standing, but denying it, defending it, or insulting our intelligence by acting like we're still fooled loses much more.

◆   ◆   ◆

Don't volunteer information the doctor does not require.

People use the doctor's ear to relieve anxiety. They believe Doctor's Privilege is all encompassing and failsafe. It is not. H/s is not your priest, bartender, best friend, therapist, or hairdresser. If you do bad things, the doctor is not there to soothe the pain in your soul and make you feel good enough to do more. H/s isn't fascinated or fulfilled by helping, and certainly doesn't see these deeds as earning you special attention. The actual "privilege" applies to medical conditions. Although there is room for interpretation the law is closer to the opposite: One must report a crime. You may be aware that doctors can face charges for failure to spot and report child abuse. The parent may be the patient; the law recognizes no privilege.

In the prison where I work I treat people charged/convicted of major crimes. I do not know any legal details of any patient. It is irrelevant that I can treat a murderer as objectively as someone who simply disturbed the peace: It can't be proven if a claim of prejudicial treatment is made. Like anyone else, a doctor is supposed to report an unsolicited confession to pending charges. If a confession must come out for accurate reporting of what happened for medical purposes, then things get more vague. Prosecution and defense attorneys have informed me differently—I guess law is also more art than science.

A patient must exercise judgment. Suppose your sin was trespassing, If you must say so to give the doctor an idea of where you were so h/s can diagnose an unusual toxic reaction, then confess. If you think getting a cut bandaged allows you to get a DWI homicide off of your chest with no repercussions, think again.

Never lie. If you weigh your health against your legal status and decide to withhold information, report that you can't say certain things and let the doctor figure out where to go from there.

Do not look for support in your legal cases/business/domestic arguments, etc. The doctor is supposed to be supportive of your cause and people generalize the "health cause" to all causes. People delude themselves that the professional, calm demeanor indicates the doctor sees no great sin in their wrongdoings.

If nothing else, stories of wrongdoings make you less likeable. Save them for a psychologist. If you are reading this book, you want to be treated as a person rather than as a medical condition. If that person is detestable, then either the doctor treats you as a bad person or heads back to treating you as a pack of symptoms. Being treated as a person brings with it the responsibility for what kind of person comes across.

◆   ◆   ◆

If a doctor doesn't seem to be supplying a time for questions, then the question should be, *I have some questions, when can I ask them?* If you don't get a polite, helpful response, you probably should be looking for another doctor, because it may be a waste of effort to try to get what you need from this one.

Be self-vigilant. If you feel ignored after being told there's no time to keep answering the same questions, be aware that h/s did not refuse to answer questions. Be sure you are not reasking the same thing and very sure you're not fishing to change the answer.

If you repeat a question for clarification or for a deeper explanation, you may want to point that out. You might have to ask where you can read more in-depth or for more basic background information.

Many people "machine gun" questions. If you are scared you'll forget one, write them down. If you constantly spit them out as you think of them, then you aren't paying attention to the answers. The questions are for show, but a commitment to do the work of understanding isn't there. If you aren't listening why keep answering?

It's sometimes an outright attack, like a quiz show: *Time's up next question, BZZZZZ you lose.* It can be a quest for openings to whine and complain. It can be the pent-up urge to ask questions exploding out on the first receptive doctor. The barrage is sometimes asking for easier levels, down to preschool. We can't give remedial shoelace tying classes.

And the Number 1 reason for the barrage: The answer is longer than the question and people want an equal part in the conversation. A barrage of questions is a more subtle method than debating the answer or adding stories, often from people least able to concede they are trying for equal time. Remember that it is not a conversation, it is an opportunity for answers.

Prepare your real questions in a short, intelligent form. Listen to answers. Only talk if you don't grasp a part of the answer. Be an intelligent student and the doctor will want you to hear the sound of h/h voice.

Some comedians rush to get the next joke out "in rhythm," even if the audience is still laughing. This trains the audience to see laughing is an interruption, and they'll politely refrain. The quiet, stodgy atmosphere will soon stop people from finding things funny. They'll feel the act is bombing, so it is. Similarly, if you overtalk the doctor, the reflex is to stop interrupting your questions with answers. Next thing you know, your act is bombing.

◆   ◆   ◆

If you are accustomed to special consideration due to your ailment, prepare to be just another person in the doctor's office. Everyone is sick, and some may even "outrank" your level.

◆   ◆   ◆

If the staff tells the doctor you are in some way special, that is the best start in becoming special to the doctor. There is more opportunity to "charm" the staff; if they are not overloaded, use your social skills out in the waiting room. If they are swamped and you make an obvious effort not to aggravate their stress, you won't regret it.

Word of rudeness to the staff beats you into the exam room. If nothing else, they warn the doctor. At this point playing nice is seen for the show it is. Oddly enough, a doctor can do very little extra for you if the staff is against it, but they can do many things for you without the doctor's knowing. They can often get h/h to do things h/s'd never consider doing otherwise. Oh, and forget those doctors' lists—staffs talk!

What if the staff can't influence the doctor? What if h/s's aloof or treats them like robot servants? Simple. Dump the hopeless clod and find another doctor. Some doctors pretend to be nice to patients, but if they have a bad personality it always comes out in their treatment of the staff. If a doctor is great to the staff, then no matter what h/s seems like to some patients it's just a facade—you can get through.[17]

◆　　　◆　　　◆

Ask a doctor to explain big words h/s uses. If there is resistance ask h/h to write them on paper for you so you can look them up. H/s will generally explain rather than do this. This makes you look more intelligent and conscientious about your own welfare. If the reason for the big words was to save time, then it will now feel less time consuming to use regular words. If the doctor hides behind the words or uses them for long forgotten reasons, this eases h/h around the habit. Use a pen and paper if necessary, but make it clear you are not trying to intimidate. Don't have them ready to pull out like a gun from a holster. Say something like, *Please spell that, I'll need to look it up to really understand.* If h/s really can't explain beyond tossing big words around, then you will have look them up. If they don't add up to an explanation, then it may be get-another-doctor time.

If h/s's given you great explanations, do not say you are writing down these things to look them up—that seems like you don't trust the explanation or are belittling what was done. Say you're writing it to remember it. That's a good moment to thank h/h again for the special effort. Doctors are people: Reward in the actual moment encourages that behavior, and praise is a great reward.

If the doctor made an effort but the explanations weren't good, say thanks. Add something like, "it would be wrong to take up more time, could you advise any pamphlets?" You might get more explanation

---

17.　Unless the relationship with the staff is a partners-in-crime thing. Such doctors are, fortunately, much more common on slow news days than in real practice.

right then. If the explanations remain useless, you might have to face the fact that this good doctor is a terrible explainer. That leaves you a decision to make.

◆   ◆   ◆

On a routine checkup say you feel well once, maybe add, *nothing new, no complaints, just here for a routine check.* Repeating and emphasizing how well you feel without being asked starts the doctor wondering: Are you

- scared to say something's wrong?

- seeking a good report for an impure reason? (Such as for a job application)

- in denial: This patient prevents the doctor from checking the problem. H/s ignores that the resulting good report is from ignorance and fuels h/h denial.

- hinting that you won't take bad news well.

◆   ◆   ◆

Whining complaints never end. Excess repetition makes it seem like complaining is the goal. State things once. If it still hasn't been addressed later on ask one more time.

◆   ◆   ◆

The doctor can make a human error. If you think h/s didn't realize something you said, simply ask: *Let me get this straight Doc, I should...* If the doctor corrects it, don't make a fuss over whether h/s said it wrong or you heard it wrong. If they report that what they said was correct you can ask about why it seems strange to you.

◆   ◆   ◆

Some patients keep repeating things like, *I'm deaf speak louder,* in angry, preachy tones. Truly hard-of-hearing patients pay hard attention, they keep silent to aid listening. There can be an element of "the class struggle" here, leveraging an alleged infirmity to talk down to "the man," but it's common for people to invent or exaggerate such troubles to hijack the exam.

The solution tends to be to act equally dismissive of the patient; however, if h/s coincidentally has a genuine condition, the doctor must try to point out that if they'd keep quiet for a second they might hear something they need to hear. This gets the doctor a repeat performance of the lecture.

If you are hard of hearing or have another problem be very clear about it from the beginning. Don't first bring it up as an insult later, *Don't you realize I can't hear well!* It is fine to ask the doctor to speak up or to repeat things as often as necessary, without lecturing. Some people who definitely hear what they want to hear play a game of asking me to speak up when I am already shouting right in their face. I call their bluff and advise them to go to a doctor who works with sign language: My normal voice tends to suffice after that.

I have examined completely deaf individuals via hand signals, (their) lip reading, and a pad to write down explanations. Fakers should realize that doctors are immune to plays for sympathy, and an infirmity doesn't excuse rude or obnoxious behavior. A doctor may be offended on behalf of h/h patients who have the real condition!

If a doctor says, *stop, that isn't necessary*, you should stop.[18] If it becomes necessary later, h/s can ask for it then.

When saying something went wrong do not add that you know that others had the same complaint. This lowers rather than raises the validity of your words. These reports almost always increase after being told that we'll handle it. We figure...

- You are insecure about it or outright lying, so you have to keep proving it. When we agree to look into it that suddenly increases the fear of the lie being uncovered.

- You may be complaining just to complain, and our taking care of it doesn't end your desire to complain.

- You may be angling for something and the fix is just the foot in the door, this is the shove against the door.

It's all silly, anyway: We can tell what's real. Ten people lying or one honest problem won't change anything. If we "fix" what wasn't broken and "apologize" for the inconvenience, we know: Welcome to our list. Many people honestly imagine things aren't just right, just thinking about anything will make them uncertain. We understand this. Trying too hard may make us confuse your honest uncertainty for a purposeful lie.

◆   ◆   ◆

Pleasant is not necessarily cooperative. If you are doing anything but exactly as requested, you must question how cooperative you are being. Entering with an argument is never cooperative. If whining does not sound natural, it also sounds uncooperative.

Taking a question from the case history as an invitation to ramble is not cooperation. There is a tendency to do this on the first or second

---

18.   Like stopping the exam to go through dozens of glasses after being told we have what we need on record.

question, irrelevant of what the question is. You can't pick a more effective time to make a doctor wary of talking than at the beginning. If you must say or ask something right away, first ask if it's okay. Then get right to the point. If the doctor has to stop your rambling, do not to try to convince h/h why h/s should hear this now. If there was a point, now you'd better save it; if it's that important, apologize and ask if you can just get to the point. Be aware, if it really was that important, of how foolish it is to bury it in stories: The doctor thinks this way, or at least reacts accordingly.

You can only hurt your relationship by debating a doctor's version of your history in that office. You're probably wrong; The doctor wonders if you are bluntly lying. You probably have more memory of your exam than the doctor does. That's why you're wrong. H/s's not speaking from memory, just reading the record! When I look at a record and ask if the patient followed the instructions they often claim they were never told to do this. It's rarely written down until after it's been told. In fact things that are written down have likely been emphasized more than one time: Doctors are equally "lazy" with written communication.

Patients who yell that they were never so instructed often mention the specific reason they didn't follow it, and then point out that they mentioned this back then. They'll still insist that they were never told to do it at all. You see what I'm getting at here?

◆   ◆   ◆

Drop any "it's owed to me you should be honored" attitude. It's a funny thing, but people who pay directly rarely have this attitude. People who pay their own insurance premiums don't have it much. People who get coverage through a job have it a bit more. People who get it from a government source have it more often. People who have no coverage at all do it all the time. It's a weird commentary, but the more people should be grateful, the bigger show they make of being entitled to more. Everyone may act this way sometime, but you never win friends in that moment.

Appear appreciative every step of the way. It's good advice for dealing with anybody.

◆   ◆   ◆

Doctor's tend to be defensive verbally, whether they're aware of it or not. However, because it's set off verbally, you can use nonverbal communication. If you simply look like you're inhibited to say something, or that you find something amusing, like anyone else h/s becomes curious. Do not flirt: It will make 98% defensive and the remainder will react to it literally, which is fine if you want to marry the doctor rather than get information.

Don't wear an uppity, *I know something important,* smirk. If you're not sure if you look cute or smug, playful, or uppity, then don't try to get any message across. The biggest lesson is what not to do. More is lost by doing the wrong thing than by not doing something special.

Use the unexpected: I often greet a doctor (or anyone) by saying something like, *Hail and good cheer,* rather than, *hello.* Defensive systems are not scanning for this: I have introduced an attention-getting level which h/s can't block because before h/s recognizes the attempt at "relating" h/s has already answered in a conscious way. Even if it's conscious of thinking that "he's peculiar," it's too late: H/s is already awake to my real existence and relating to me. H/s may not gush information yet, but h/s will not stop relating unless you do something special to warn h/h back into h/h shell.

◆   ◆   ◆

In a big hospital patients often feel like a piece of meat or worse—one organ is the meat and you're just the packaging. Doctors complain about resultant problems from the other end. The system does pressure things to be this way; however, it isn't all the system's fault, and that's where our tricks come in.

Don't attack the doctors. They have had it with this system more than you have and don't want to defend anything to you. To them the systems exist because of decades of financial choices by patients. The doctors are victims of spending trends of the consumers; that's you. Approach them as someone who understands how difficult this terrible system is on everyone. Approached correctly, most of these doctors are on your side against the powers that be.

◆   ◆   ◆

To every doctor there's a specific aspect that fascinates h/h and it is easy to get them to talk if it's involved. It is easier to find what this is with a specialist, but it is not simply the specialty per say. H/s may find this boring in general by now, so look for something like a subspecialty within it.

◆   ◆   ◆

Orders are not polite: As a doctor, when I want you to do something for my comfort I will say "please"; if I want you to do something for your comfort (or necessity) I may not. There are reasons not to say "please," such as speed of response when it's crucial. "Please" can invite a discussion or conversation at a bad time. Don't look to find reasons to be offended—let it go. Curb your urge for ego fulfilment or feeling like you've "won" and understand what you want and how to get it. Misunderstanding yourself is your biggest communication obstacle.

One inappropriate goal that will sabotage your chances is the need to change the doctor. You aren't a *Ghost of Christmas* changing *Dr. Scrooge* for everyone; you're a customer making sure Scrooge provides what's coming to you. The doctor's behaviors and defenses are there for a reason and will only change slowly as patients and the system appear "safer."

◆   ◆   ◆

Much of what I have said for patients is good for doctors. I've observed these patient-doctor dynamics, and many doctors confirmed that these affect them. This doesn't mean the average doctor or the super-busy "star" doctor has given them any thought. Being aware that you, doctor, have developed behavior patterns is a start even if you disagree with my details. These insights can only be debated if you come up with your own.

We now have the problem that all patients have. Doctors are doctors and see themselves as the expert in the medical room. It is hard to get some of them to accept that they need improvement or outside help in so fundamental a skill as talking. Still, read on for some...

Suggestions for Doctors

7

Suggestions for Doctors

The medical profession does acknowledge the need for better communication. Courses for doctors do exist. From all reports they have a long way to go. It seems the general format is to take words like *patient, doctor, sickness,* and *treatment* and substitute them for words like *executive, meeting, proposal* and *contract* from similar courses for corporate (or other) settings. Meanwhile, the complaints from patients on the matter haven't diminished.

Many doctors have taken communication courses and felt these had nothing to offer. Their attitude isn't arrogance, it's realism. I can understand why any doctor who wanted a course that took h/h real world into account would become quickly disillusioned.

I have seen this in other fields. I have watched people solicit students who had no intention of performing into comedy or improvisation courses to help them in their regular lives. I learned improvisation alongside a few students like this. Nobody actually engineered courses for the different purposes. They simply marketed the regular courses to a larger "audience."

On the other hand, I have heard good things about some programs that didn't exist at all even a decade or so ago. Actors do play patients with specific symptoms to train doctors.[1] I have heard they give valuable training to future doctors both in diagnosing and bedside manner. Foreign students seeking American licensing must pass a clinical skills test using such actors. Making this a general requirement has been dis-

---

1.   Always on the medical cutting edge, Seinfeld did an episode about this.

cussed. Although it is a start, actors who may make the viewer believe h/s is seeing the real thing may not see (and hear) things the way the actual patient would. Their reactions are guesses at realism based on guessed emotions. A real patient may react to very different cues. Letting the actors grade the doctors is a copout on the part of the system: Instead of trying to understand communication, setting parameters and a system to teach and test for them, they are putting the onus on actors who are not medical experts or patients. They don't know what's in the patients head, just what they seem like to watch and what symptoms they have according to the lists they memorize.

I see the actors having far more use in training doctors to get things out of the patient for diagnoses than for training the doctor to soothe, calm, and instruct the patient. The battle has begun; however, the recruitment drive may be the biggest problem.

Let's divide doctors into five groups when it comes to the communication problem:

1. Doctors who deny a problem exists or don't care. I haven't found very many of them.

2. Doctors who truly communicate well. They also appear to form a very small minority.

3. Doctors who believe every other doctor has the problem, but that they are the rare exception who communicates well. This is a surprisingly large group.[2]

4. Doctors who believe they communicate well enough. Finding a way to improve is not on the "to do" list. Together with those who believe they communicate well these seem to account for the vast majority of doctors.

---

2.   And every patient is sure h/s is a fabulous communicator, which is at least as far from the reality. Me, I'm impossible, which keeps me on my toes...

5. Doctors who acknowledge their personal needs for improvement.
    A small group.

Getting more doctors to move into the last group may be the biggest
battle. For any doctor reading this, perhaps reading such a book is a
sign that you are moving in the right direction. Even if you disagree
with everything else I write, acknowledging your need to improve personally is the key step.

Medical communication problems involve more than just the doctor and patient interaction. The doctor-staff interaction is in need of
some upgrading, as are the doctor (and staff) supplier/administrator/
third-party interactions.

Even the doctor to doctor interaction needs serious help. A communication course to train practitioners to give each other a better feel for
a case would be invaluable in hospitals where shifts take over for each
other. Obviously, it would help if time and coverage were provided
when shifts switch so doctors could converse and possibly visit specific
patients together if necessary. This would alleviate many problems of
three-shift days, where, for instance, an emergency patient becomes a
case from scratch three times.

There is an assembly-line quality to task assignment in a hospital
where each employee does the same thing for many patients. At no
point is the doctor employed to spend a lot of time talking. The hospi-
tal/insurer systems would have to change to get anyone-in-the-know to
talk to each other and to patients in a superior fashion. Hospitals could
possibly then schedule doctor time for just talking with patients and
bill for it, and for communication support staff.

Everybody claims to believe that the job of the medical system is not
to "process patients and count results," but to improve the patient's situation. Insurance companies and other institutions spend millions
advertising their adherence to such principles: The money would be
better spent integrating it into their daily practice. Doctors, insurers,
and patients have to learn that the job involves getting the patient to
take care of him/herself with proper effort and comprehension. Sur-

geons especially must self-monitor for viewing care as something *I do to them.*

A week does not go by in which a story about surgery on the wrong leg, or organ, or the wrong patient does not come to my attention. Generally, the news source mentions many complicated proposals for preventing such mishaps and many reasons that these can't be done presently. Try this technology: Provide one human being on the surgical team who comes to know the conscious patient at earlier times and greets said patient[3] before sedation begins, or at least looks at the patient's face to see who the unconscious *person* actually is.

Doctors would also benefit from a communication course geared toward the corporate world. When you are "employee X7B59," it helps to speak the language of X7B59's world.

Control issues

People do not take well to any suggestion of losing control. This reality is exacerbated logarithmically[4] in this age where we are trained to be hypersensitive to such things: We have trouble taking orders from people who pay us to do so, so what chance does anyone else have? On the other hand, actually taking responsibility to think and plan is another story: We want a benevolent force to control us and things around us all while allowing us to maintain our illusion of being self-independent.

---

3. A stranger greeting a patient won't do. Patients answer to and confirm the wrong name all the time. Some do it on purpose to be taken now and figure they'll correct the identity mistake when a good opportunity arises, others are simply "tuning in" only to the fact that someone is offering to give them attention. They don't register the name called, on some level they just mean "yes, I'm listening Mr/Ms. Voice," not "Yes, I'm the one you are asking for." If you call him/her by "the wrong" first name several times they keep "forgiving" you without mentioning it!

4. A real, real lot!

Doctors must take charge and possibly even give orders. Patients know this. We can't assume it follows that they remember to accept it. Knowing it's coming makes patients see it in everything a doctor does. Doctors may tighten up inside while facing minor medical mutinies throughout everyday. Some might go numb and treat patients as a bunch of results and numbers.

Doctors have to become aware of every dynamic to nullify their own tensions and reactions: They must review all patient behaviors with some "how does that make me feel" work.

Patients will also actively do things to have some control. For instance, patients lie or hide things in their history to keep the doctor from having "the advantage" of that knowledge. In refractions it is common for a patient to deny having glasses several times, only to pull out many pairs at the end. They feel they have controlled things because we couldn't use these as a guide to get the findings or to make sure the findings don't match exactly so we can make a sale. They will generally demand a complete retest taking these into account.

When things are this blatant, I find being equally blunt in return works best. I deliver a prepared speech telling him/her that h/s is trying to control a professional, which is a foolish undertaking: A pro can toy with you on h/h own turf; if the pro can't be trusted, this would only make him/her angry. I unemotionally inform him/her that I take no offense at the fact that I have obviously not yet earned h/h trust, but because h/s needs a doctor with whom h/s feels comfortable, h/s should go find one and drop me.

I have delivered this speech a hundred times, easily! Every single time the patient begged me to take him/her back, and most became model patients. These people referred friends. Some have told me that they've treated other doctors differently since that and over time those doctors have related to them on a much better level.

I've never found another doctor willing to talk quite like this. Pity; people trust people who *politely* put them in their place when it's needed. After this speech I become the great and wise doctor they trust—To put it bluntly, blunt works. Doctors are extrascared because they're supposed to be superproper. They forget that truth is always proper and bluntness is a sharp[5] tool (to be used surgically).

Doctors should learn something about presentation and delivery. In writing, especially comedy, it is understood that it isn't so much what you say as how you say it. In performance this goes further: It's how you sell it. In any field the great successes are often not the brightest nor the best, but the natural salesmen. These message spinners have a sense of how to say the same thing and have it sound much better.

There are ways to tell a patient about their condition, the need for referrals, surgery, and the like, that set the patient in a preferable frame of mind. For a simple example, how do you tell patients that their insurance is not accepted here? Not the way most doctors and staffs "sell" it.

The problem generally is that the insurance company hasn't put the doctor on it's panel. Human ego puts everything in the "we weren't rejected, we turned them down" form, so doctors/staffs say, *we don't take your insurance.* This has the "side effect" of making "we" the ones to blame. Explanations are demanded, but they're never fully accepted. Yelling and fighting may ensue to make you take their insurance this time or "make it up to them" by seeing them gratis. Tell patients the truth: *They don't take us.* It's so simple it's beyond belief how effective it is at reducing wear and tear on the staff.

If you'd like the insurer to accept you well, as long as your staff takes the abuse for the insurer, the insurer isn't getting any message. I've stepped in and told patients, "I understand you're anger, you're wasting it on our staff. Please, save it, stay angry, and call your company."[6]

---

5.   Fresh off the press new oxymoron, "sharp bluntness."

6.   Doctors have pointed out that sometimes they do turn down a coverage plan because it pays super low and late (if at all), while demanding impossible extra services. The reality is that they do refuse to use you in a reasonable manner. Tell the company your rules for proper payment; They will turn you down. If you turn down a reasonable company for your own peculiar reasons, then you may have to say, "We don't take them."

On the topic of how to say things, the right pronoun can save a lot of grief. When stating conclusions say "I," as in "I'm finding evidence of infection." When stating medical fact say "we," as in "we feel that this is handled best this way..." It psychologically shuts the door on openings to start trouble. When it's borderline, if you can say "we" without sounding obnoxious,[7] go for it. With a patient who appreciates anything personal say, *I find this one works the best in such a situ...* For those who like to debate detail and fact say, *we find...*

On occasion, a patient reacts to something like, *we do this all the time for such problems* by saying, *who is "we," I've never seen your partner...* I explain that I am referring to doctors in the field, not in this room. That does wonders. This patient might have attacked things from my experience as opinion; now it is fact. Saying "we" instead of the less humble "I" has the psychological power of writing: If it's in writing, it must be true!

It is also useful to know when to say "we" in order to include the patient. For instance, instead of "I will test you" say "we will do the test." This works better than long speeches to get a patient to accept some responsibility for their care. It also makes them feel less like a helpless victim of painful things. Never say, "I will drill your teeth" or 'I will give you an injection" or 'I will do a glaucoma test on you." Instead try, "we will fix your teeth," "we will take care of the injection," or "let's get your glaucoma readings." Anxious people are more likely to react to tone and manner than to (the comprehension of) literal detail.

I use my own tricks to minimize the problems. For example; instead of just saying that a problem is not related to, but actually predates, an injury for which they may be trying to collect compensation, I first predict information based on this: *From what I see you could not have had an eye exam in 15 to 20 years, if ever.* They'll reply, *How did you know*

---

7. One is accused of lacking humility for using the royal "we" too often. It is actually egotistical to say "I" when it really is "we" (in the field...).

that? I get to say, *Because you could not have checked and missed this old condition.*

One more example: When I say "relax, it looks fine" I might add, *to the limits of testing and from the description of symptoms so far, but that doesn't mean to ignore a new or worsening symptom.* That usually works magic. Some anxiety stems from a fear that they'll feel things after I said, "we're done," and anxious people always find trouble. Showing I understand that *being done* isn't written in stone let's them relax. Worriers imagine less problems, nonworriers are less likely to ignore a real problem.

◆   ◆   ◆

Some doctors might be good talkers, but on-the-job circumstances change everything, including the motivation. I probably have more trouble than most, my natural speech has been compared with "ZIP files" of normal talking. Perhaps I have an advantage of being attuned to listener feedback for translating my internal speech to comprehensible speech, a skill all doctors suddenly need on the job.

Some doctors do need to learn to talk and others need to learn to explain, but many need to learn to listen and to ask the right questions. Doctors, however, mostly need to be re-motivated. They need to want to talk and to *resist the resistances.*

There are two kinds of resistances. There are the admitted things like fear of saying something that will come up in a suit, fear of wasting too much time, fear of wasting breath on patients who won't get it anyway, fear instilled by rules from the employer, and fear of being uncovered as an incompetent.[8] In certain cases these are exaggerated in your mind; in others, the pressure is very real. It should be pointed out that even when it is real, such as with an employer who monitors per-patient time, you can always improve within the constraints. There can

---

8.   Then take more courses! D'oh…

almost always be more and better dialogue while working without moving into extra time.

There are also the resistances of which you are unaware, such as habits from med school days or subliminal reactions to a patient. If you can't name the resistance or if it makes little sense, the best way to get over it is to just talk more. Nothing will happen to you. It's easier than dieting; it's more like learning to eat more: It's habit forming.

There is one odd resistance; the resistance of making a patient too much of an individual. Except in rare television drama moments where adrenaline charged doctors beat off the forces of death, the cool, calm, collected, "automaton" doctor who never panics has some advantages. On the other hand, involved, interesting conversations draw important information out of your patient. Everything gets explained better, compliance is more likely, and unfounded patient concerns are alleviated.

Conversing in such a manner will make the patient more of an individual. There might be concern that this will come at the cost of the doctor's calm objectivity of detachment. That would make little difference. First of all, if it happened, you can bow out if you ever feel "too involved." (In an emergency you must pull yourself together anyway. Heck, if an emergency happens to somebody near you, they are most likely also to be somebody *close* to you.)

Think about it: With real emergencies brought to you there is no time for any connection and it's likely that many of the patients aren't conscious. Patient-perceived emergencies like broken arms are too mundane to threaten your calm. You do need the patient more calm and cool to avoid the only thing that can go wrong: losing control of a panicking patient. Getting your interest (attention?) level more in line with that of the patient would help. A real conversation would raise yours and moderate h/hs. This works better than fake, babyish (patronizing?) "cooing" about how "okay" everything is.

I do not engage in long-term treatment that can end in an emergency situation such as with cardiac or cancer care; however, I have heard of numerous cases going better because the doctors and staff connected with the patient.[9] I have never heard of a surgeon fumbling because h/s got too close to a patient. Surgeons have become distraught over losing a patient as if they'd lost a close friend. There is pain in becoming closer to people whose days can only be stretched so much. TV likes to show doctors who can't function for their remaining patients; indeed, I have heard of one or two doctors who simply had to call it quits.[10] I have heard many more stories about doctors who "messed up" because they had become uninvolved to the point of distraction.

I see doctors inadvertently get close to patients and have so few problems that it never registers that they became close. They'll burn up on adrenaline for the patient, yet their denial of the reality keeps them detached when it comes to nervousness. It's more the adrenalin of aggression (anger) than of fear.

No matter how close a patient becomes they are a patient first, and a doctor's frame of mind stays correct. If they were cured and became a regular friend for years and then became ill again, it might be different. Even then, when closeness blurs a borderline call it is easy to say, "You were very ill before, I want to be overcautious." Every single time another doctor told me that h/s stays detached on purpose, it clearly rang more of excuse than of reason.

Any doctor who does not actively work to keep patients from becoming individuals should check him/herself for any behavior that

---

9. I do volunteer performances for hospital patients. I have done more than 150 comedy shows at Sloane Kettering Hospital starting in 1993. There, I am a comedian; the doctor part is unmentioned. I have a unique opportunity to watch the dynamic and hear what patients think. Maybe not all of their observations are correct. That doesn't always matter. Doctors should be more aware of patient perceptions.

10. It's bad enough that patients accuse you of thinking you are a god. Don't punish yourself by judging your performance as if you should be one. People have to learn that the doctor's job involves more than saving those who can be saved; it includes improving the quality of life for those who can't be saved. Doctors really have to learn this, beyond paying lip service to the concept!

was developed along such lines, or behavior that was trained-in by mentors who behaved this way.

A bigger fear is that these conversations will exacerbate the long, rushed day. In reality they remove much of the tension of the day, so it becomes a bit less of *something to be survived*. If you still just don't like breaking down certain barriers, talk more anyway. I talk to people to entertain myself. We may really connect through the conversation, and walls may collapse as far as what they'll share, but not as far as becoming closer as individuals. People such as these have a name: audience members. Converse to keep from being bored—patients are the audience. You don't have to be entertaining—the act of the talkative, attentive doctor is always a big hit.

Valuable information comes out of patients in conversation. When doctors feel there is something not being said or being altered, they try to get the patient to talk. This starts as questioning in a "playing *Sherlock Holmes*" way, but it becomes more of an interrogation of a captured enemy. Great interrogators don't interrogate, they converse. More information flows when someone who is withholding it is off guard.

Some doctors have moved away from conversing with patients because they really don't want information from patients: They don't trust patients to do anything properly on their own behalf! Although many doctors acknowledge that they do many things to get patients to follow instructions due to this "crisis of faith," few realize how insidiously the attitude has spread to every aspect of their patient interactions.

Often this starts from a rationalization of why they should put up with so much abuse: A doctor may harbor a sense that people are like children whose transgressions must be ignored because they are not capable of responsibility. Some put it into humanistic terms, such as *I feel it is my responsibility to care for every patient to such a level where they're human foibles are accounted for in the treatment course*, but they're saying the same thing. One doctor may feel, *Patients are terri-*

ble, you can't trust them to do one thing for themselves. Another may say, *Patients are all wonderful in their own ways, it gives me joy to handle every detail for them.* There's a feel either way that people must be handled like children rather than relied upon.[11]

♦   ♦   ♦

A doctor is supposed to act "professional" in the face of extreme rudeness. This is only asked of people who are supposed to be above the fray, such as clergy, referees, judges, people who deal with children, and police. Only clergy can compare with doctors in performance, but they're supposed to be emulating saints.

A case can be made as to why all the others should be above it all, but why should doctors turn the other cheek to misbehaving adults? It may have something to do with making people feel welcome to medical help despite themselves: Because medical care is considered too important to be denied, there are people who figure they can behave as they like and still get the same care. There is no actual law against doctors being rude in return. Things should be handled as when dealing with the public from any business standpoint. Smile through a little abuse, but don't encourage or permit any escalation of it.

A patient should never be allowed to believe that obnoxious behavior was okay because it caused no obvious reaction. It tends to be all or nothing from h/h vantage point: They do something and the doctor ignores it. They do worse and, if anything, the doctor looks more professional while restraining normal human emotions. This patient will escalate to obscene levels of abuse to get the desired reaction, if only to

---

11. And, unfortunately, they may be closer to the truth than if they assume adults are adults. Antibiotic-resistant germs are often the fault of patients! No amount of emphasis gets them to keep on the medications after they feel they're okay. That leaves only the few strongest germs to live on and produce an extra strong colony. Now the patient self-prescribes the leftover drops. Repeat this cycle a couple times and voila', superbug.

confirm success at bothering someone. The doctor finally says this will not be tolerated. Then the patient acts victimized.

Rude patients should be made to understand that outward appearance of calm or not, the doctor can deal with a person in any fashion that they deserve. Doctors should let patients know early that rudeness and aggressiveness on their part are noticed and not tolerated. At the cost of a few patients acting wounded and saying you overreacted to nothing, almost all the real problems will disappear. People who meant no offense are apologetic for the misunderstanding. Acting offended is a defense of people caught in the act: If you play along and apologize, remember to watch them.

Early intervention keeps the question of when to take the kid gloves off from coming up very often. This will eventually put a different ambiance on all patient interactions. Doctors who never realized that they "clammed up" for most of their patients will be much more open with the vast majority who have never been very rude or threatening.

Words mean only a fraction of the total in delivering a message. People react to perceived emotions. If you act angry, people think they did something wrong. If you don't, then their transgressions are your fault. If someone is dropping heavy things where your foot is and you calmly tell him/her to stop, h/s actually has to subdue anger. In their gut they received no message of anger from a victim, so there was no incident. In that gut they are mad at your interruption. Many people disassociate: They're logically sorry, yet they know they are angry. They just aren't sure what about you is making them angry.

I normally manage to look exasperated with rude patients and the message is clear: *Enough is enough. From now on it's fast-food-style care for you. Tell your symptoms into the clown's mouth then pull around to the side.* People with reason to be defensive get very bothered by a little reaction. They may complain to the staff or administrators, but there isn't anything specific to mention. Most are too wary of being asked why they thought a facial expression was a reprimand of them because they are aware of the answer: They recognized it as a one because they knew they had earned one.

Doctors who have tried letting responses show more freely in their expressions and manner agree that it works. If you insist on maintaining a non-emotional professional level, at least show the effort of controlling the reaction. Freely showing reactions actually makes it easier to hide what has to be hidden, such as your reaction to a potentially serious finding.

Many rude patients get this message without realizing it, so they "comply" without getting defensive. People treat people with respect when they show they demand it. As for the few people who won't give up the attack and just get angry at the message, treat them as they deserve: Everyone will be better off if they take their "business" elsewhere.

◆   ◆   ◆

How do you talk to a patient when there is no right thing to say? Everyone else can avoid this person, but not the doctor. Even a clergy can eventually let it go if the patient doesn't want to talk. To make matters worse, the doctor must talk as one who can help while also following the conflicting "rules" everyone is trying to figure out for talking to a person beyond help. If that's not enough, anyone else might be forgiven for saying the wrong thing, but the doctor is held to a higher standard. In truth, the close friends of the patient have the most "expertise" for the matter of knowing how to talk to this person.

The answer is simple. As far as feeling helpless, you are only helpless if you view your job as being to cure every sickness. If you view it as doing whatever you can for the person with the sickness, then there is much that can be accomplished for the person, even if the disease must ultimately take this patient (or their limb, sense, organ...) from you. I cannot train anybody with a sentence or two of instruction to sense what can be said (yes, it's the same sense I use to define humor), but I can give a simple guideline. Say something! Avoidance by the doctor is the single worst thing. A patient senses that h/s scares off the doctor. Whether it is a fear of being near incurable disease, death itself, the feeling of helplessness, or failure, the patient is affected. You'll never say the right thing if you don't try. As long as you try to say the right thing, taking it the wrong way is the patient's doing. H/s was going to take nearly anything the wrong way, they are not worse off for your trying. Accept that, feel no guilt, feel no tension, "coldly" let their words pass by you, forgive them any unpleasant feeling you can't prevent, and keep talking. That's the only way to hit upon the right thing.

Workshops and Rehearsals

Should you treat the patient as an individual, or treat a patient as a case? Of course I am not seriously posing this question as if it's up for debate, it's a trick. In the first half, "the" patient sounds personal, in the second half, "a" patient is being discussed clinically.[12] Humans overreact to such minutia, the meaning does not change at all and "a" is probably the slightly more accurate choice by the rules of English. However, a person hearing "a" feels the writer has an impersonal view compared with a writer using the word "the."

A writer truly taking a more personal view might be more likely to choose the word "the," but the writer would also have lots of time and chances to experiment and choose. I thought about it—I'm a writer[13]. For people talking it just comes out, so it is important to train to make certain choices. Such training is technically called "rehearsal." Playing doctor is a role that should be rehearsed as any other. Sales and some other corporate departments accept this. Doctors, police, and teachers are among the many others who should wake up to this concept.

---

12. How fascinating and unfortunate it is that the term, "clinically" has come to mean "in a cold, detached, manner!"
13. Will somebody please tell my editor to stop laughing and finish editing the book.

In simple read-the-book form I have much less specific advice for doctors than for patients. For one thing, as a doctor I have far more experience with patients than being a patient. Fear not patients—doctors have more to do. Doctors should take actual workshops. Communication is an instrument that needs lessons and practice like for piano. Courses covering theory and facts are of limited use to say the least; something more like acting classes with rehearsals is the ideal.

Thinking like an actor will add one other dimension to the doctor's communication abilities: The nonverbal communication. Most real interpersonal communication takes place on levels other than the words; the words are often just filler. Performers are trained on other levels. This is especially important when dealing with patients who have limited abilities. The problem goes beyond getting the message across, it is the lack of feedback to keep us going. We must become more aware that we (all humans) need feedback, which some sick people cannot provide. I cannot begin to list the stories from patients, relatives, staffs, and even doctors who don't understand where things went wrong that point to one thing: Most of us don't realize that we mindlessly display terrible reactions to the lack of normal feedback!

I'd better explain. Nobody likes to be interrupted, but we expect it. In fact, we can't talk without it. If we go on too long without being interrupted we check for attention and begin doubting our ability to keep the people interested. Some listeners are good at physically showing interest and some listeners, who may be used to having people silently riveted, are used to sensing the difference. Most people feel they've lost the audience if they don't hear interrupting sounds. At least in person they can check for things like eye contact, although insecurity will eventually cause them to rate the quality of the eye contact; if your expression doesn't change enough they begin to feel you are sleeping with your eyes open. This is far worse on the phone. In fact, I have my own little reply ready when my attention is challenged because I am listening for too long: (you want to know what I'm doing...) "This is the sound of me listening."

Performing stand-up at hospital shows one faces an audience that might be somewhat sedate, due to being sedated. At such times I advise comedians to keep going, the silence does not necessarily mean they are bombing. It takes a few times to get over the instinct to bail on the material and try something different. I don't mention that with more experience one learns to tell the difference between a sedated but appreciative crowd, and a sedated crowd that is also bored.

Everybody wants the emotional security of responses that prove we are being heard, even though our thoughts are to wish these interruptions would stop. We will naturally focus on sources of such reinforcement. In other words, with a perfectly intelligent but highly immobilized ALS[14] sufferer, we will instinctively turn to h/h companion and speak about h/h. Doctors must rehearse communicating with the right person and get over our reactions to the lack of the responses that they cannot provide. This happens with very old (and young) patients, mute patients and many others. When speaking through a translator we must always focus on (and, at least some of the time, make eye contact with) the patient.

Doctors must also learn the importance of the emotional component from the theatrical world. Yes, some people have psychiatric problems in which there are emotional disturbances that require treatment. Unfortunately, doctors tend to view all emotional reactions as symptoms to be treated. Few doctors would ever admit to this, but most act this way at some point. When you tell somebody that they have a dreadful disease, you must learn to deal with an appropriate response. It is part of your communication assignment as a healer. The knee-jerk (trigger-happy?) reaction to add, "and I'll prescribe some antidepressants and sleeping pills to help with…" is a sign that it's the doctor who can't deal with the reality.

It is also a matter of self-delusion. We don't want to feel helpless, but when we cannot soothe a crying patient we feel that way. We can't offer an instant guaranteed cure, so instead we focus on their reaction:

---

14. Lou Gehrig's Disease

The problem isn't that they are ill; rather, it is that they feel bad about being ill. Let's drug them out of this state! By ridding them of this normal (healthy!) reaction a functioning system has been messed up and the complication of their pharmaceutical picture has begun.

As doctors we all signed on to help people who may ultimately be beyond medical help. The job is to help them as much as possible anyway, not to drug them into acting like things are okay so we don't have to feel uneasy.

One very easy thing for any doctor to do is to get a better grasp of the patient's perspective. I highly advise taking every opportunity to be the patient of a doctor who does not know that you are a doctor. An added bonus will be that if you manage to hide that fact you will probably be a better patient for your doctor. It's not only on TV that doctors make the worst patients.

There are several reasons for this:

- Doctors with a disabling condition feel displaced; on the wrong end of the conversation and trying to get back "home."

- Doctors have major trouble with the control issues, they are used to treating other doctors as peers.

- It is hard to nudge doctors into behaving because they are immune to the tricks that make patients comply and feel good about the treatment.

- Doctors know that symptom "X" may mean condition "Y," especially if followed by symptom "Z." Obviously they will experience "Z" no matter what.

If you can find these behaviors in yourself it will do more than help you control them when you are the patient: It will help you recognize them and your reactions to them in your own patients. That will go a long way to being able to remedy the situations. By the way, in the last example, the solution might be to come clean and in robotic fashion state, "Okay, I'm a doctor, so I think I experienced Z, but I was waiting for it long before that!"

◆   ◆   ◆

Maybe a few doctors reading this book will realize there is a need. Maybe they'll try to integrate some of the simple things this book recommends, and perhaps they'll consider a workshop. They can ease their own lives and just maybe help their patients.

◆   ◆   ◆

Some basics have been covered. Maybe in the future I'll have a chance to discuss the ever growing supply of anecdotes and some of my "personal" things. Of course, I am expected to end with a summation and some fancy ending prose, but first comes the section I've been waiting for…

8

Open hailing frequencies Or Why humor?

Where does humor come in? Universally declared to be the best medicine, laughter, of course, is a great healer—unless it is used near anyone who is sick! *It's just not right to laugh; this is serious stuff.*

I am often asked whether I "behave" in the office or if I can't stop some of the zany stuff from coming out. Although I am "on" twenty-four hours a day, it's still a show—I never have a problem stopping it. But why would I? In some ways I can go farther in the office than I can onstage! In the act the audience won't buy something if it seems too detached from normal reality. In the office the "audience" buys everything because their doctor is really doing it. It's their problem to convince other people that they have a doctor like that.

That brings us to the more philosophical part of the equation: Is this the place for such a comedic persona? My answer is not the obvious. I am not going to write that I think you can use some humor. My answer is that it is actually the only proper way. Everybody employs inferior or inappropriate "attitudes" because they can't do the humor with enough margin for (potentially offensive) error.

As I have probably mentioned at least once, humor is a medium to deliver the message. Any message. I could just as easily say that at a sad occasion it is inappropriate to break into song, yet every type of sad occasion has it's music; for example, a funeral has a dirge. Just being funny and laughing as if in celebration can be wrong because the wrong content is used as the message. It would be like doing a song and dance from a big, upbeat Broadway show at a funeral.

Just as any message can be put into lyric and melody, any message can be packaged in humor. Gallows humor anyone? A side order of nervous laughter and little asides? Perhaps the problem lies in thinking that laughing is in and of itself an emotion. It is not. The emotion it is confused with is a happy or even joyous one, but the tie is not absolute. Festive people laugh easily, but angry people laugh a lot, and anxious people may laugh deeper when the source of their anxiety is attacked with humor. They are not necessarily happy even if their anxieties are soothed for a moment. Scared people naturally joke to ease the stress on the system, but they remain scared. Sad people do some joking; depressed people often make jokes about how bad their situation is or how unworthy they are.

We all have many opportunities to deal with an upset person and take their jokes as a sign they are better. That may be a bit premature. We sometimes chime in with supportive jokes having taken their lead. Some of them appreciate the help working this out; others get mad. They ignore that they have been making jokes and see your ability to make the same kind of joke as a sign of not taking things seriously. They are confusing your use of humor with happiness, your match of their humor with the humor called levity (lightness).

The beauty of humor as the package for a message is that it can package the highest percentage of content as subtext. Any part of the message that the listener isn't ready to deal with has in effect never been given. It's as if they "decode" only what they can accept. The rest is unheard or dismissed as just in jest. It also softens the hard parts. To a degree the medium is also a message. The message of this medium is to take the best outlook considering the situation. That's why gallows humor is universal to bad situations.

As a simple example, let's say I have to inform someone that they might need an operation. I want them to understand that they must see the specialist, but I don't want them so alerted that they panic and avoid the specialist. I also want to emphasize the relative safety and capability—I am sending them to see if they need surgery because I believe the surgeon is able to help them. When the patient says something to the effect of, *So you think they may have to do surgery and cut open my eye!* I would reply, *It's not like their taking a rusty blade and hacking away; it's not the eighteenth century or even the 1950s. Hey, it's not even the primitive 1980s.* Depending on the level of the reaction and interest I might continue and supply more real information contained in increasing levels of jest.

Here's another example. If I tell someone who seems doubtful or anxious that h/s should *let it run its course,* I'll add something like, *I know, I know, that's what they told the guy in "Alien" and "Its" course ran right through his innards eating all the way, but this is slightly different...* The fact that I didn't wait for the question removes the possibility that the question makes me at all uneasy. The humor itself belittles the situation. Not the medical situation, mind you, but the situation of this person being anxious over it; however, it does not belittle the person for being anxious—after all, I anticipated this reaction so it must be normal. At most I am having fun with the nature of being human, not with this patient personally.

You say you didn't know so much information was included in such little jokes and their positioning and timing? Sure you do—that's why they work; but you might not be aware of having that knowledge. It's all happening where it counts, viscerally. Psychologically. Emotionally. Few people have it analyzed to this degree, but many people with top-notch delivery[1] know it in their guts. Almost everyone has the integral knowledge to understand the message, but only a few have enough integral knowledge to be great at delivering the message.

The way I look at it, the more somber the doctor the worse the situation seems. Such a doctor makes good news seem serious and neutral

---

1.   Don't go running to ask someone down the block just because h/s performs comedy. I said "with top-notch delivery." And even then some are just good at copying the delivery of others.

news seem worthy of panic, but truly serious news can seem no different. A cheerful doctor keeps a patient from panicking, and can control an irresponsible patient with one "serious" sentence. If h/s can lighten the mood, it doesn't mean h/s's insensitive to my plight; it means h/s doesn't find my plight to be such a, plight.

Let's take a quick look into this world of "visceral messages." As strange as this sounds to many people, it is the truth behind almost all person to person communication. People do very poorly with facts, but are excellent with the communication of emotion and nuance. Even those who are accused of being blind to it are generally quite the opposite: They are hyperaware of it in order to know when to keep the shields up. Part of those shields is having zero reaction to such incoming messages.

In an argument it rarely matters what is said: The more emotion behind it the more the other person is pushed away. At best any reasoning in the words is used to rally the person saying them. Very few people have the intelligence to take in facts and re-evaluate and alter an opinion: Arguments go on because neither side has enough intelligence to be able to lose!

If you state with no anger to someone that their statement is wrong, you have still challenged their intelligence and authority. Logic is irrelevant—that person is reacting to an inferred[2] challenge of a personal nature. To give in on the facts is not simply to say you had the better facts or even that you have more knowledge or intelligence in general, it is to defer to your authority. Point out an error in fact as a question and it will psychologically be taken as supporting their authority, so only the facts matter. In fact, to demonstrate their authority they like to play with their own facts. For example:

Person A: "It's 65 degrees today."

---

2. Because it is not always meant this way we can't say it is implied. The listener, however, almost always "infers" it this way. Few people are aware of this as they say it, but hearing it would offend them the same way.

Person B: "It's only 55"

Person A: "Shut up you idiot—I know what I'm talking about"

or

Person A: "It's 65 degrees today."

Person B: "Is that what the news said? Do you think it feels like only 55 though?"

Person A: "Yes, yes I do. I believe the report is off. I'd say it's more like 56 or 7"

We discussed an interesting version in the previous chapter: People are always fighting to be heard, but then being heard isn't enough: They assume you will interrupt; therefore, if you don't you must not be listening at all.

Patients must realize that they affect the doctor in the same way. For instance, it is not unusual for a patient to enter the exam room saying something like, *The thing is,* in a stern or angry tone. Make sure of your tone. Even the words here are visceral dynamite. They are not the start of the conversation; they are the middle. This person has been rehearsing a confrontation in h/h head and is preemptively striking to prevent reactions to the obnoxious things h/s has considered doing.

We are always tuned-in to visceral messages, we must become aware of the messages we send and of the (perceived) messages to which we are reacting.

◆   ◆   ◆

People confuse "serious" with a lack of humor. This is because we use the word that way for lack of knowing the proper word. If I said give me a word to describe a person with no sense of humor, the single most popular answer by far would be "serious." When someone is seriously angry at you and about to knock your head loose h/s will spew a lot of jokes and put downs. This humor means they are very "serious" about what they plan to do!

"Serious" on my part means accepting that you and your problems have substance and value and that I will deal with your case carefully. Patients confuse this with a somber demeanor and want it right up until I show them better. Doctors are afraid to use humor. In truth, even patients who say they want it as part of a warmer more personal doctor-patient bond generally want it for a warm greeting and that's it.

The reality is, integrating humor takes a lot of skill—a "sense" of humor in that truest sense: a keen sense of how and when and how much. There are patients who are looking for any reason to complain, although, fortunately, humor doesn't seem to be on the list of what they look for. They can go ballistic, however, if humor is used to assuage another complaint. Some people are simply antihumor, but it doesn't take a pro to sense this and tone things down to comply. Almost any patient can become upset over humor if it isn't delivered the right way. Some patients will get too logical in retrospect: *Hey, h/s made me laugh at my problems and deal with them without panicking; humor is supposed to be inappropriate; h/s didn't respect me and my serious condition...*Because of this each practitioner should integrate humor gradually, and always err on the comfortable side.

Unfortunately, despite decades of everybody paying lip service to the value of humor as the best medicine, it has never lost one drop of the prejudice against it. It is segregated. It is only allowed in situations where everything is fine and dandy and happy—exactly where it is least needed. We segregate it from our problems even when we do use it to battle the problems. We go to clubs to have a professional do our jokes for us or we watch shows that let us escape rather than deal with our problems. The problems are just as upsetting when we return. Even parodies of our problems become an escape rather than a helpful perspective.

The time for laughter is when dealing with the problems. It is your shield. Do you know why a bully makes fun of you when h/s attacks?

To belittle you. In one way or another you are their problem. Hurting you doesn't change that; belittling you is the more important point. It emboldens them for the fight. There is a reason that they'll force you to say that you agree with the insults as part of the beating: They need to be reassured because they fear you or what you represent to them.

The first step to being able to tackle any problem is to find the strength[3] to laugh at it. Whether you believe in the power of laughter per se or not, few will debate that mental state has a lot to do with recovery. This is so even on a physical level because the brain is a chemical factory; an immune system battery. A happy brain is like a little locomotive that *thinks it can.*

There is a lot of back and forth going on here. I am selling the value of humor and its appropriateness, yet mentioning that there is a mind-set against it by doctors, patients, and even people who think they are staunch advocates of humor in health care. It should be done, yet even if it helps it can cause trouble if the wrong person picks up on it. The truth is it is a tool that never backfires when used correctly. If humor seemed to help but the patient later stopped to decide that humor was still inappropriate, something was done incorrectly. The usage wasn't smooth: Maybe the doctor laughed too hard at h/h own joke. That's unprofessional for a comedian, but it can be downright offensive from a doctor. Maybe h/s paused too long to enjoy the "audience reaction." If you don't move on you give people time to review and that's where complainers can take notice to start trouble. Beside, the joke should have been for the patient's benefit. The doctor should look pleased if the patient says, *Thanks for making me feel good with the little talk we had,* but h/s should not seem quite that pleased directly for getting laughs.

Humor is nearly entirely avoided under the general principle of *the less you do the less can be done wrong.* I think patients understand without being told why doctors might turn off this aspect of their personal-

---

3.   I actually see it as finding perspective more than finding the strength. Perspective gives you the strength.

ity; however, if doctors would take baby steps, everyone can find their level and improve things around the office. It certainly helps the staff if the doctor at least uses some levity to set a less stressful tone.

I use more humor on the job than others are likely to ever use. In two decades I have never once received feedback to the effect of, *funny guy, not a good doctor.* Some people just look at them as separate things: Personality and professional ability. Others realize that the humor actually helps in some ways. Some seem to have a reverse rationale, *He must be good to get away with being funny; he doesn't need to act formal like all the others.* Even the occasional unhappy patient has never complained about the humor. The truth is, patients who are going to be unhappy no matter what show their cards in plenty of time to remove any excess or risky humor (or any personality at all) from the proceedings.

Humor defers to the patient (as long as you don't pause to revel in what a great performer you are). It defers in the most important way, to h/h existence-as-a-person. H/s's not a slab of meat, h/s's someone worthy of being amused, worth the time to relate to above and beyond the exchange of cold facts.

In comedy, it is better to be liked by a crowd than to overwhelm them with talent. In medicine, the doctor who earns the patient's faith is a more successful healer than the doctor with the most knowledge.

We hit a *Catch-22* here. People want to relate to a human doctor while being treated by a godlike doctor. A deity you can relate to on a human level implies a mortal god, an oxymoron. Couldn't a genuine god, however, seem to relate like a human while remaining godlike? A god could. Few doctors can do it well. Such a god would likely use a very powerful tool to do this, one that causes most doctors to tremble in fear. You got it on the first guess: Humor. Most doctors probably have the misguided belief that humor would ruin the godlike aura because it might seem unprofessional. In truth, to "the gods" everything on mortal earth is of small consequence, nothing is serious, humorous would likely be their default operational mode.

There are times when the patient should take the first step. Make a little joke and then your doctor doesn't feel the pressure to be super-proper. Even if h/s is incapable of adding any humor the lower pressure removes one reason to avoid talking. The doctor may not realize it, but without the fear of saying something the wrong way, more words will flow. Beside, you instantly become the patient people instinctively want to help. You're not whining; you're strong. You're considerate. You tried to make things lighter instead of playing for attention as a victim.

◆   ◆   ◆

Being a doctor is a lot being a comedian.

- You take your best guess and then the better you sell it the better it works.

- If a joke doesn't work, you examine every aspect of the writing and the performance to improve the act. It is said: We learn the most from our failures in everything in life. It is best not to ever mention that to a patient.

- Few comedians are really actors, but they often play them on TV. Doctors are not really gods, but they play them on the job.[4]

- They both get to say, *You say it hurts when you do this, then don't do this;* however, only doctors get to hear a patient respond, *Why not?*

- They are the only two professions in the world that you must keep secret from strangers or else you are guaranteed to be asked for a freebie. *Really, you're a comedian, tell me a joke. You're a doctor? Say, I've been having this problem....* As a comedian I reply, *You're confus-*

---

4.   Or as we have learned about there not being any magic moment that a student feels h/s has become a doctor, every doctor at some point has felt, *I'm not really a doctor but I play one in this clinic.*

ing me with a comic, I don't tell jokes. As a doctor I point out that the equipment needed to answer their question properly is at the office. Some will push on with, *Just give me an idea of what this is and what to do with only the exam you can do without equipment.* If it goes this far I get to answer, *But there is one piece of equipment at the office we need, it's indispensable, unless you're paying in cash so I won't need to authorize any coverage.*

- Both are obsessed with lawyers. Here's a question for extra credit. Who said the following, a doctor or a comedian? *People pay a lawyer hundreds of dollars an hour to hear them complain that a doctor didn't spend enough time talking to them at no extra charge. And to top it all, they pay the lawyer more for the extra time it takes to complain about the cost of having had their life saved than they paid to have their life saved in the first place!* Oh, sorry, trick question, it was said by a lawyer but overheard by a comic.

- Both take a stand against Dr. Kevorkian, the suicide doctor. And both secretly wish he was around every once in a while.

- Both would love to hit the HIP center with a wrecking ball then send them the bill for a "HIP Replacement Procedure."

- Neither can read their own notes.

- Lots of people think most of them are never funny.

Okay, and here's the big difference between doctors and comedians.

- Everyone who has a joke that isn't good enough to tell to their friends is sure that you, as a professional comedian, will appreciate it and need it for your act. I at least get to respond: *I have more than enough material for the act but I do seem to be running out of fresh procedures to perform on my patients. If you've come up with any creative little methods I'd love to expose my patients to good, folksy, cutting edge nonwestern medical techniques.*

The following is a classic old joke but it fits in with this book far too well to ignore.

THE PATIENT

A woman called Mount Sinai Hospital. When the hospital switchboard answered she said, "Mount Sinai Hospital? Hello, darling, I'd like to talk with the person who gives the information regarding your patients. But I don't just want to know if the patient is better, or doing like expected, or worse. I want to know all the information there is to know about the patient…from top to bottom…from A to Z!"

The voice on the other end of the line said, "Would you hold the line please, that's a very unusual request."

Then a very authoritative voice came on and said, "Are you the lady who is calling about one of our patients?"

The lady answered, "Yes, darling! I'd like to know the information about Sarah Finkel, in Room 302."

To make a long story short the doctor gives the woman all the information she asks for. At the end he asks her how exactly she is related to Sarah Finkel?

"Oh, I am Sarah Finkel. You know, the one in Room 302 to whom you never tell nothing."

To round this section out, here is my favorite joke that I made up that came true several years later and then again several years after that…

The job of everyone working in the correctional system is to help the inmate break the cycle of returning to prison. As an optometrist I feel I do a big part. If I can get the right glasses onto someone who has always had trouble reading, working, or even getting around, then h/s has a much better chance of not returning. H/s will be more productive, fit into society, and next time the opportunity comes up, h/s'll see the cops coming.

Or, as it turned out, see enough detail to know that the guys coming are wearing uniforms!

That's The Ballgame

Some people have a gift for charming anyone, or at least for getting them talkative. It can be enhanced and maybe even taught, but that would be for a long-term live workshop. It should not be faked. For our immediate purposes it is more important to do nothing wrong to send the doctor (or patient) into a shell than to try to become the great communicator instantly. This leads to perhaps the most important point to emphasize.

Doctors are human. That's the main message. If they sense you desire something of them, they dole it out in small little rewards…and that's if they don't take it the wrong way and get defensive. Without knowing it the vast majority of humans who sense they have the upper hand in a relationship play hard to get. If they sense disinterest, then they crave interest. It is why playing hard to get works.

That is, as long as it doesn't seem like you're playing hard to get! One must seem truly hard to get: If one is obviously playing games, then despite being called names relating to insincerity (sleazeball, slut, etc.) the truth is that one has simply become unattractive. To play means to pretend, which means it isn't true. It shows a need to work to ensnare the very person you are pretending to push away. This need shows you don't believe you are that desirable. In the doctor's office you're very attempt to act like the great communicator or charmer can doom the attempt. It shows an effort. That effort is to get more of something, in this case communication.

The trick is to play hard to get without being caught. Doctors have complained to me of patients who listened only to be polite, but who seemed to have more interesting things to get to. When I pried the doctor invariably realized h/s had fought for that patient's attention in every sense of the word, by talking and giving more of themselves.

Doctors are from Earth and that's how Earth people are. The Earth patient sensing this became bored with this doctor who needed h/h attention.

It is good to remember doctors' humble Earth origins to guide everything you do in dealing with them. No matter what kind of front they present they react the way you probably do. The more people I speak to, the clearer it is that whether you are a mechanic or a waiter or a delivery person or the CEO of a large conglomerate (and even more so, h/h secretary), people do the same things to everyone who gives any form of service. Doctors may experience more exaggerated forms and they must have a longer fuse simply because the word "client" has been changed to "patient," but it's the same thing. The difference is that a deli owner empathizes with the bank teller when h/s sees the same abuse. When I show how the same things occur in medical offices they are shocked; not shocked that it happens, but that they have seen it often yet avoided taking notice. They had been refusing to see doctors as people being taken advantage of, to the point they may have become rude or abusive themselves.

In general, whenever an opportunity presents itself let it be known that communication is part of your doctor/hospital/HMO choice. This is more important for the long run than for you in the moment. It seems everyone complains about this, but few people let the powers that be know that it will affect pocketbook decisions. Let the business end get the message en masse.

◆   ◆   ◆

Being from Earth a doctor is subject to the same ups and downs, moods, personal and family problems, and responsibilities as you are. So far as I know nobody has formed any kind of priesthood of celibate doctors or a monastery type of hospital…despite some having a monastery aura of an oath of silence.

Never forget that even within h/h professional domain the doctor is not a godlike Lord of the Manner. H/s has many orders, rules, regulations, obligations, and pressures. H/s is also constantly evaluated. In the worst forms this means doctors avoid the neediest patients because they or their technique will lose some type of support based on statistics.

Even the government actively supports bad treatment due to ignorant but good intentions. Grants are awarded for things that work. Most money for funding breakthroughs goes to proposals that are easy to "sell" to the funding agencies. The more they sound like something the agency already understands, the better. This means the vast majority of funding intended to spur breakthroughs—from government or otherwise—goes to proposals for ever-so-slight variations on what everyone else is already researching.

Exceptions still occur, so occasionally a promising technique somehow manages to get researched to the point of being implemented. In that case, things get even worse. If I take 100 incurable patients and miraculously save 10 of them through an ingenious breakthrough, that's a 10% success rate. If a butcher of a doctor down the block picks out 100 easy to cure patients with earlier, milder versions of the same disease and nothing else to complicate things and then through h/h general lack of "excellence" loses 20 of them, well h/s has an 80% success rate. Guess who's getting a better rating! To insure that their new technique receives good evaluations, the doctors who have the technique that might save a hopeless patient are the least likely people to agree to treat h/h. They need to prove their technique through a high success rate, more than other doctors do: They are forced to screen for the easiest patients—the ones who don't truly need this special help.

Doctors face many pressures. If you are ever trying to convince a doctor to "do the right thing" and ignore a pressure, the last thing you want to do is to start by challenging them on the points that already make them nervous. Even if you could wave a magic wand and make all doctors perfect, including in their communication skills, there would still be problems as long as there is no perfect system to keep every single other patient honest, sane, polite, and sincere. Your doctor and you are not only from Earth, you're still on Earth. It's a jungle out there. Mere mortals, even doctors, have to be cautious.

◆   ◆   ◆

I have discussed putting some personality into any verbal greeting. It has occurred to me that I have preferred ways of ending things. Basically when the exam is finished but the patient just wants to hang around I have several "fallback" ways of indicating we have to end sometime. If a patient in the hanging around mode asks if there is anything else left to do or discuss I might say, "As the *Yankees* say when *Mariano*[1] comes in, That's the ballgame." Even *Met* fans appreciate the line, they know what a good closer is worth.

The line had to be given a rest when Mariano had that unfortunate experience to end the 2001 World Series. A couple of months later a situation was begging for the line and I decided it was time. To make the lawyers out there happy I did deliver it with the proper legal disclaimer regarding the minor exception in the bottom of the ninth of the seventh game of the World Series, but the point's still the point.

Having my line back caused me to think about the nature of a closing line. Onstage you want to leave on a big laugh for reasons specific to the craft of comedy. Some comedians actually reverse engines and discuss something serious right before the ending joke to leave a *take-me-seriously* impression. If an act employs this h/s really needs a solid finale joke to always leave them wanting more. There are no related reasons to have a big ending as a doctor. So why did it seem so important?

That it works is unquestionable. Some patients enter the exam room and state *I've heard you're really good.* Some say that's why they asked to

---

1.   For those who don't know he is a relief pitcher famous for coming in and shutting the opponent down to end the game.

see me but others make it clear they were already here when earlier patients said these things. The single biggest factor in how many patients go out and compliment me is the *closing bit*. Patients are much more likely to spread the word if they leave wanting more. The question is why it works so well.

It's important because although first impressions impress, last impressions last. A lot of great communication and effort to deal with a patient as a person can be ruined by having a patient leave feeling h/s was rushed out because the assembly line of care had moved on to the next patient. The mood is different when ending with a joke. More significantly on our good old visceral level is the fact that the very words informing the patient that the end is here are delivered as a joke. Even as things had to end time was still taken to say it this way instead of just the blunt stark facts. Effort was made to give this one last confirmation that you have been dealt with as a person or maybe even that the doctor enjoyed chatting with you and is just as unhappy to have to move on as you are. The line probably comes out better the more true this is, when it isn't true no such line may be forthcoming anyway. Some people will not budge unless told to leave in clear terms and they are never the ones you'd want to hang out with any longer.

Anyway, as the Yankees say when Mariano…

0-595-27200-2